Praise for *Weight Management for Your Life*

"This book debunks myths about weight loss, empowers people by giving them the information and tools they need to 'change the things they can change,' and, most importantly, sets people up for success."

– Louise Lettre-Klingensmith, LMSW (clinical counselor, Columbia, SC)

"At last, a weight management book that calls for personal responsibility and empowers the reader to do it 'your way.' I recommend this book for all health care practitioners and individuals frustrated in dealing with weight loss."

– Edith Hessel, RN, MSN, cPNP (Washington, DC)

"*Weight Management for Your Life* presents a complex area of research thoroughly and clearly. It makes a case for common sense long-term lifestyle change in a way that empowers and encourages people to compassionately engage with themselves, develop a plan, and carry it out. ...It is exceptionally well written, researched, and well reasoned."

– Patricia Feigley, MSW (clinical practice of psychotherapy and yoga instructor, Columbia, SC)

"Dr. Goldman acknowledges the importance of integrating one's feelings with one's thoughts and behavior. ... Activities for the reader and Internet support are additional tools making this self-help book all you wanted to know about weight loss."

– Linda Meyers, M.Ed. (St. Louis, MO)

About the author

Dr. Goldman received his undergraduate education at Yale University, medical training at University of Missouri Medical School and Cleveland Clinic, and psychiatric training at University of North Carolina, Chapel Hill. As a professor at the University of South Carolina Medical School he authored more than 25 articles in the professional literature and has written three book chapters.

Weight Management for **Your** Life

TEN STEPS TO PREPARE YOU FOR ADOPTING A HEALTHY LIFESTYLE

Charles Goldman, MD

ISBN: 1-4196-9256-9
ISBN-13: 9781419692567

Visit www.weightmanagementforyourlife.com, www.amazon.com, or www.booksurge.com to order additional copies.

For George Vaillant
Whose teaching and research inspired me and so many others

CONTENTS

Preface

Have you ever said, about managing your weight, "I know what I have to do, I just need to do it!"? I must have heard some version of this statement hundreds of times.

Most people know about eating less and exercising more, and also know it is not easy to do on a consistent basis. I appreciate this dilemma as well as anyone, which is why I decided to organize what I have learned over the years in the format of a self-help book.

As a physician for over 35 years, most of that time practicing as a Board Certified psychiatrist, I have witnessed hundreds of people struggling with managing their weight. My experience as a psychiatrist is relevant, because much of my practice has consisted of helping people become more aware of their options, recognize and eliminate self-defeating patterns, develop skills that will help them maximize their strengths, and learn to make decisions that are in their best long-term interest. I have never had much affection for the "victim role" that some people prefer, and have worked hard to increase feelings of empowerment in myself and others.

I have observed the weight loss and exercise self-help literature for decades, and have come to the conclusion that most of it is misleading because it panders to our desire for a quick and easy solution to a difficult problem. Few books about weight management deal with the subject of self-empowerment seriously or in much depth or breadth. My objective in writing this book is to summarize relatively simple ways to begin to overcome the problem of eating too much and exercising too little.

I said the solution was simple, but that does not mean it is easy. There is a big difference between the two concepts.

The solution is simple because it only involves engaging one's mind to make a commitment to eat less and exercise more. To maintain your weight, calories taken in must be in balance with calories expended through metabolism and activity. More or less eating, and more or less activity, affect the ratio. All of the variables are under the control of voluntary behavior. If more calories go in than out, you have weight gain – only 100 extra calories a day can add ten pounds in a year! Weight loss results from changing the ratio in the other direction: reducing calories in and/or increasing calories out. Simple.

At the same time, using your mind (or "willpower") to change the way you eat and move can be very difficult. Most people do not really know how to fully engage their mental and emotional resources in a way that will get them through both the initial difficulty of changing behavior and the lifelong commitment it takes to maintain the healthy behavior.

Who this book is for

This is a self-help book for people who want the basic information and skills necessary for choosing a healthy weight range and maintaining it for life. It is for people who suspect or know for sure that the power needed to adopt a healthier lifestyle will come from within themselves, even though they may need help and support to fully tap and focus that energy. Please use it as a source of encouragement and guidance to assist you in becoming healthier and improving your quality of life.

Weight Management for Your Life does not feature a diet or weight-loss plan in the usual sense. It contains no recipes, recommends no products, nor does it offer a "quick start" program. Instead, it will give you the tools you need to choose a way to eat and exercise for life, and reading it will improve your ability to evaluate diet and exercise programs that are being marketed through books, magazines, ads, and infomercials.

The advice in this book is not intended for people who have a severe eating disorder, tend to be underweight, or have extreme obesity and are looking for a way to lose 100 pounds.

On the other hand, please do read this if you are mildly or moderately overweight, if your weight is in a healthy range but you are concerned about possible weight gain in the future, or if you don't really know what a desirable weight range should be. This book will help you determine whether you are ready to make a commitment to proactive lifelong weight management and, if not, what actions and decisions might bring you to that point. Also read it if you are concerned about the health of a friend or loved one who may be overweight.

Although this book is based on my many years of experience with weight management as an individual, family member, and health professional, I wrote it from a holistic perspective. It is my strong belief that weight control, though extremely important, is only one part of a lifelong commitment to health and happiness.

How to use this book

The book is organized so as to make the difficult tasks involved in behavior change as simple and natural as possible. All you need to do is read the introduction and the next ten chapters. Each chapter is organized so you can very quickly discover "**what you need to know**" and then explore the topics in **more detail** in the rest of the chapter. The small numbers (superscript) that appear in the text ("footnotes" or "endnotes") refer you to reference material or additional information arranged by chapter in the final section of the book.

After reading the **ten steps** in Part 1, use the **easy action steps** in Chapter Eleven to begin to apply what you have learned. These action steps are designed to help you translate the content of the reading into behavior, one step at a time. Additional chapters in Part 2 give you even more detailed information than the previous chapters. If you do most of the exercises in Chapter Eleven, you will be able to say with confidence, "I know what I want to do, and I am doing it!"

PART ONE

Introduction

**"Whether we live to a vigorous old age lies not so much in our
stars or our genes as in ourselves."**

– George Vaillant[1]

WHAT YOU NEED TO KNOW

Whether we live a long and healthy life and feel satisfied in old age is at least in part determined by the way we think and what we do to help ourselves. A reasonably healthy lifestyle, including weight control, exercise, moderation in drinking and no smoking, can make a huge difference in our long term health and happiness. Adopting a positive "glass half-full" attitude, valuing lifelong learning and interests, and nurturing supportive relationships are the other keys to aging well. The ten steps in the chapters that follow this introduction will give you the knowledge you need to make significant changes in behavior in order to better manage your weight and generally improve your health and happiness.

MORE DETAILS

How to be "Happy-Well"

To "see the glass of life as half-full, not half-empty," and to "understand how to savor joy and how to turn lemons into lemonade," according to Harvard research psychiatrist George Vaillant, are the thinking patterns of people who age successfully. In his book *Aging Well* he describes in detail the long-term outcomes (at ages 70 – 80) of three groups of people who were studied with thorough evaluations every few years from youth through old age. The research subjects were 724 men and 682 women, 63% of whom lived to old age; all were initially included in the research because they seemed "normal" and were free of any obvious illnesses or disabilities.

Vaillant writes about factors that seem to predict which research subjects turn out to be Sad-Sick (including dead) and which Happy-Well. One description of the Happy-Well group highlights their "learning to live with neither too much desire and adventure nor too much caution and self-care. ... Rather, successful aging means giving to others joyously whenever one is able, receiving from others gratefully whenever one needs it, and being greedy enough to develop one's own self in between."

After reviewing the data on all 1406 subjects Dr. Vaillant was pleasantly surprised to learn that most of the significant predictors of positive outcome were things we have some measure of control over:

> "The protective factors ... – a stable marriage, the ability to make lemonade from lemons, avoiding cigarettes, modest use of alcohol, regular exercise, high education, and maintaining normal weight – allow us to predict *thirty years* in the future. ... **The good news is that most of us – if we start young and try hard – can voluntarily control our weight, our exercise, and our abuse of cigarettes and/or alcohol, at least by the time we are fifty**. And with hard work and/or therapy we can improve our relationships with our most significant other and use fewer maladaptive defenses. I do not wish to blame the victim, but I do want to accentuate the positive. **Whether we live to a vigorous old age lies not so much in our stars or our genes as in ourselves**."[2]

The results of these studies and Dr. Vaillant's thorough analysis give a huge boost to those of us who believe that *our conscious health-related decisions* are extremely important in determining how well we live and enjoy old age.

What is most relevant to weight management about Vaillant's work and the other research on lifestyle choice is the message that one can *learn* new ways of thinking about one's situation and can *practice* new behaviors that will result in a happier and healthier life. I have found this to be the case personally and in my psychiatric practice.

This book provides a guide to get you started in changing your lifestyle. The approach involves education and behavior change. In my experience, people have only bits and pieces of the knowledge they need to successfully alter their lifestyle. We are bombarded with information and misinformation, opinions and gimmicks, and this can be overwhelming. The following chapters present ten basic steps to prepare you to evaluate the information you come across and, more importantly, help you engage the power of your mind to improve your life.

Chapter 1

Step 1: State a reason to change your behavior

"We have goals because that's how our brains evolved: the people without goals became extinct because they simply could not compete."

– Marvin Minsky[1]

WHAT YOU NEED TO KNOW

Weight control, or lifelong weight management, for most of us, requires work. We will not do the work unless we are convinced at a deep level that doing so will get us what we clearly want. Therefore, we need to put into words the specific reason(s) we desire to maintain our weight in a certain range and state this as a goal or goals.

There is a long list of proven health problems associated with being overweight, and avoiding these problems is reason enough for many people to control their weight. Each person should study the list in this chapter and focus on the specific health problems that are most worrisome for them. Also, other, more personal, reasons for controlling weight should be clearly spelled out from the start. This list of goals, or reasons for committing to hard work, will be very important to refer to at times of discouragement or frustration.

MORE DETAILS

Health benefits of controlling weight

Although some classify extreme obesity as a disease, I think of being overweight as a risk factor, not a true disease. Some "experts" view being overweight as a symptom of deeper psychological troubles, and view overeating as a form of self-medication.[2] I think that can be true for some, but there is scant evidence that overweight people generally have underlying psychiatric disorders.

Some eating disorders, such as bulimia and anorexia nervosa, and some forms of morbid obesity, *do* follow the disease model and are not addressed in this book. "Morbid obesity" or "clinically severe obesity" is defined as being 100 pounds or more over ideal body weight (or having a Body Mass Index – BMI – of 40 or higher)[3].

Health problems that have been linked to excess weight, and may be at least partially prevented by controlling weight, include:

- Pre-diabetes and type 2 diabetes (sometimes called: insulin resistance, impaired glucose tolerance, metabolic syndrome, or borderline diabetes) – this potentially devastating disease is clearly tied to being overweight (especially abdominal obesity). Weight loss has been shown to reverse or prevent progression of the disease, at least when it is not too severe (see *www.diabetes.org/risk-test.jsp* to find out if you are at risk).
- High blood pressure/Heart disease.
- Stroke.
- Certain types of cancer: men who are obese are more likely than non-obese men to develop cancer of the colon, rectum, or kidney. Women who are obese are more likely than non-obese women to develop cancer of the kidney, uterus, or breast (postmenopausal). Breast cancer patients who are overweight risk higher mortality. Esophageal, pancreatic, gallbladder, thyroid, and liver cancers have also been associated with obesity.
- Dyslipidemia/High Cholesterol (for example, high total cholesterol or high levels of triglycerides).

- Osteoarthritis of weight-bearing joints (a degeneration of cartilage and its underlying bone within a joint).
- Depression.
- Sleep apnea and other respiratory problems.
- Gastro-esophageal reflux (GERD; "heartburn").
- Infertility.
- Urinary stress incontinence.
- Menstrual irregularities.
- Lymphedema.
- Gallbladder disease.
- Nonalcoholic fatty liver disease (NAFLD).
- Pulmonary embolism and deep venous thrombosis.
- Some types of hernia.
- Dementia/Alzheimer's disease.

Some research indicates that elevated waist circumference (Men: equal to or greater than 40 inches; Women: equal to or greater than 35 inches) is a more specific risk factor for some diseases, such as prediabetes, than weight or BMI. An increasing waist-to-hip ratio may be a better indicator of coronary artery calcification than either waist circumference or BMI.[4] Therefore, weight distribution, as opposed to weight alone or BMI, must be taken into consideration; belly weight (abdominal obesity, "visceral fat," or "central adiposity") is of most concern.

Making a commitment to losing weight, in my experience and based on my bias as a physician, makes sense only in the context of also deciding to be healthier in general. Certainly preventing the health problems listed above, or reducing their severity, is important.

Turning wants into goals

At this point, I must make an important distinction between "wanting" something and deciding to get it. We constantly want things, external (a new sofa) and internal (be nicer to our parent). We may desire to be rich and famous, or strong and sexy, or to live a long life free of disability. These desires and wishes are merely thoughts and feelings that might or might not lead to actual decisions to go for them. When we really want to achieve something, we make it a goal. Goal setting need not be a formal or labor intensive process, but the main goal or goals you come up with pertaining to weight management should at least be written down.

For most people reading this book, there is no doubt in their mind that they want to lose weight and maintain a healthy weight range. Probably, they have stated this many times in the form of a New Year's Resolution. It can be useful, when translating a resolution or wish into a goal, to phrase it in a way that has strong, personal emotional meaning. Goals related to weight loss might include "look and feel my best," "lose weight to avoid a knee (or hip) replacement," "keep a steady weight so I need only one wardrobe for each season," "get off medication for hypertension (or diabetes, etc.)," or "worry less about my weight." People who actually *do* something long term about their weight usually eventually spend less time and energy worrying about food, eating, and weight control. The same is true for exercise. Replacing worry with goal-directed action is a good rule of thumb for many issues in our lives.

There are so many potential goals we can have that we might be overwhelmed, so some people find it useful to relate them to an overarching **personal mission statement** based on core beliefs and values. If this interests you, use your favorite search engine on the Internet and look up "personal mission statement." You will find many helpful, free websites that assist you in coming up with a meaningful statement or list. Before writing your statement, think about your values, and also your strengths, joys, and vision of how you would like to be remembered. For me, a very brief mission statement works best.

Simply stating a well-considered weight management goal (or goals), and making a sincere commitment to carrying it out, can be done without much fuss about where it fits in terms of other life goals and directions. Some people move directly from declaring their goal to action; they "just do it!" That is certainly an example of exercising willpower. But most of us need more guidance than "just do it." That's what the rest of this book is about.

In the book *Cognitive Behavioral Treatment of Obesity*,[5] the authors emphasize the importance of their patients choosing other personal objectives besides weight loss. These are termed the *primary goals* and "commonly include a desire to improve appearance (particularly to modify shape), a desire to improve self-confidence and self-respect, a desire to be more active, and a desire to improve health."[6] During the weight stability part of the program, when most patients are discouraged by their failure to lose as much weight as they had hoped (or frustrated that the rate of weight loss has slowed), the *primary goals* become the focus of treatment. In most successful weight management programs, reminding people *why* they wanted to lose weight is critically important.

The following case example, which will be continued in Chapter 7, describes a person in the earliest stage of deciding to adopt a healthier lifestyle.

Case example: Sue, part 1

Sue is a 31-year-old woman taking a serious look at her life for the first time. When she turned 30, a friend gave her the book *Aging Well*, by George Vaillant, and Sue took it as a joke. But six months later the friend, a nurse, urged Sue to read the book, because it really was written for young people and had a lot of relevance. Now, having read the book, Sue wondered about what the rest of her life might hold in store.

She was reasonably happy and had lots of friends who enjoyed her company. She knew she was thirty or forty pounds overweight and had half-heartedly dieted, usually every January. She worked hard in following the diets (whether they were low carb, low fat, or high volume) because she always performed well, if only to reassure herself she was smart and not lazy. But the diets soon bored her, and she always regained the five or ten pounds she lost, plus an extra pound or three, and by summer was preoccupied with avoiding the beach and having to wear shorts or a bathing suit (Heaven forbid!).

She looked at her parents' lives and felt anxious and sad. They were good-natured people, and not miserable, but her dad, now in his early 60s, had already had five-vessel coronary bypass surgery and her mother, at 57, was obese and struggled to control diabetes and its various complications. Sue herself already had pre-diabetes, borderline high blood pressure and arthritis in her left knee. She knew there was more she could do to be healthier, but where to start?

In her job as an administrative assistant, she was the go-to person in a crisis. An expert multi-tasker, it seemed she could handle anything. But when opportunities for promotion or career advancement came along, somehow she was passed over, or never bothered to pursue the opportunity.

Her steady boyfriend for three years, Larry, a shoe store manager, was a comfort to her. They shared similar interests in movies and dining out, and spent most evenings on the couch watching TV and snacking. He, too, was overweight, and refused to consider joining her in any kind of fitness program when she brought the subject up (usually after some talk show host interviewed a weight loss expert, which seemed to happen weekly). Larry also showed little interest in marriage or having children with her. She did not mind, because "if it ain't broke, don't fix it."

Sue considered herself a well-adjusted person with a good sense of humor and the ability to enjoy life and roll with the punches. She knew a lot of people with far worse problems than she had! After reading Vaillant, though, she wondered whether she might be a "glass half empty" person. When something bad happened, she would blame herself and ruminate about it for a long time. When something good happened, she would assume it was luck and, even if she were complimented for the way she brought a good result about, she would shrug it off. She never thought she deserved the good stuff. This realization, that her attitude was not really as positive as she had assumed, bothered her more than anything else.

Sue truly enjoyed doing things for others and received a lot of pleasure from their response to her helpfulness, though of course she never expected gratitude. But now, really for the first time, she wondered, "Am I neglecting myself?" This question felt greedy and selfish, yet ... Vaillant had a point, she thought, when he wrote "successful aging means giving to others joyously whenever one is able, receiving from others gratefully whenever one needs it, and **being greedy enough to develop one's own self in between**."

Stigma

In order to understand Sue and her situation fully we must view her objectively, but also will no doubt sympathize with her as she struggles to find a comfortable place in a culture that devalues overweight people. No discussion of overweight individuals would be complete without mentioning the problem of "social stigma." Social stigma is negative bias toward someone because of their 1) external appearance, 2) presumed deviations in personal traits, or 3) membership in a race, nation, or religion that is considered by the dominant culture to be deviant. The first two parts of this definition apply to people who are "overweight."

People are stigmatized because they are considered unattractive, even repulsive, by the trendsetters in a culture. This form of stigma is independent of the presumed cause of the deviancy, and therefore doesn't take into consideration whether the condition is an affliction (e.g., leprosy or cleft palate) or brought on by the person's own behavior (e.g., dressing like a "nerd" or neglecting dental care). Obese people are devalued in our culture because they do not match the current "ideal" of a person who appears youthful and fit (people we now call "obese" would be considered sexy in some cultures today, and would have been envied at some other points in history).

In addition, because of our growing fear of overpopulation (global warming, etc.) and the reduction in available physical environment and natural resources, there is even more pressure on people to not over-consume, take up too much space, or leave too large a "carbon footprint." Overweight people, of necessity, use more food and energy and take up more space than thinner people.

People are also stigmatized if the larger society blames them for their own predicament. To the extent that we believe obesity is brought on by lack of self-discipline, this belief adds to the stigma, and presents a problem for scientists and health practitioners who treat obesity as a health problem that can be alleviated (at least in part) through behavioral interventions.

There is evidence that some degree of stigma is actually helpful in reversing the public health problem of childhood obesity. A controversial program in operation for decades in Singapore requires overweight school children to participate in exercise classes and special dietary programs, thus stigmatizing them in the eyes of their normal-weight peers.[7] The program has been successful and may be a model for what could work in other cultures, and many of the children grow up to be adults who are grateful they were in such a rigorous program. Still, many feel they were psychologically harmed by the stigma they experienced as children. There are no easy answers.

This book, to the extent that it focuses on what individuals can do to control their own weight, adds to the perception that self-discipline plays a part in what we weigh. As a physician and researcher, I am troubled by this dilemma and do not wish to become part of the stigma problem. However, I strongly believe that honesty and a search for what is true or valid are more important in the long run than being "politically correct" in the short run.

Some scientists studying obesity bend over backwards (it seems) to claim that people have no control over what they weigh, and congratulate themselves for their role in fighting stigma. I sometimes wonder whether they are being truly objective or are biased in their own way against looking carefully at all potential factors which influence weight. The rush is on to find a gene or hormone to explain obesity, and to find a pill to "cure" it. There is comparatively little basic research going on to discover how self-control works in the brain and what factors affect "willpower." In part, this bias in favor of biological, rather than behavioral, research is related to the way we fund research – through large academic/corporate complexes (looking for a quick answer that can be patented and commercialized) and through the Federal Government, which has its own corporate ties and political agendas.

I can only hope that my discussion of weight management is comprehensive and balanced, and reflects the genuine feelings of compassion, tolerance, and respect I have for people who are not considered "perfect" in our culture. My belief is that none of us is perfect, and that we all need encouragement to work on improving our health and happiness. I also believe that we have much to learn about how our brains, minds, and social networks affect our ability to exercise self-control.

Easy action steps

For specific ways to apply the information in this chapter to your life, refer to the **easy action steps** in Chapter 11. Each of the ten chapters in Part 1 of this book has exercises designed to help you apply the concepts to your specific situation.

Chapter 2

Step 2: Choose a realistic weight range

WHAT YOU NEED TO KNOW

Definitions of overweight and obesity are not standardized and not based on adequate research, so it is critically important to choose a realistic and reasonable weight range to have as a goal for weight loss and/or weight maintenance. Although weight may not be as important as other measures, such as Body Mass Index or waist circumference, it is clear that one can weigh too much in relationship to the goals selected in Step 1. Gradual weight loss works much better than rapid weight loss in the long run, and preventing weight gain, for some, is a worthy goal in itself.

MORE DETAILS

It is indeed unfair that, given the same amount of activity, some people's physiology is such that only a minor degree of overeating has a major impact on their weight, while some people can eat more without gaining weight. It is also frustratingly true that how easily we gain or lose weight varies with our age and other (e.g., hormonal) circumstances.

Despite the unfairness, I am simply defining overeating as occurring if the amount of calories consumed results in realistically unwanted weight gain. I use the term "realistically" to emphasize that our weight range goal should not be chosen arbitrarily; it must be consistent with the "set point" determined by our genetics and body type. It is extremely important, yet difficult, to remove all moral judgment from the term "overeating." It is a behavior pattern I am talking about, not a moral weakness or sign of depravity. We all overeat, and also under-eat, at times, but what I am referring to is a longer-term pattern, one that results in unwanted weight gain.

"What is a reasonable weight for me?"

A key question for weight management is what a desirable, realistic, and healthy target weight would be. Research shows that adults have ranges of weight toward which we naturally gravitate. Some people call these ranges "set points," but I believe that term implies a rigidity that is inaccurate, so I will use the term "comfort range." There is no clear-cut way to determine that range, but the upper end is probably at least what we weigh now (if we are overweight). Our choice in the matter may be limited to staying in the middle or lower end of that range. As an example, I will describe Bob's situation:

At 40-years-old, Bob was not happy with the way his protruding gut looked in the mirror when he undressed for the shower. He had an athlete's physique in his 20s and 30s when he regularly played tennis and jogged. Now, his only physical activity was golf about twice a month. Bob was six feet tall with a medium frame, weighed 200 pounds, and was starting to have pain in his knees. His wife complained about his snoring. He thought he needed to lose 30 pounds to get back to what he weighed when he graduated from college. But, after doing some research on the Internet (for example, see www.halls.md/ideal-weight/body.htm), he guessed that his "comfort range" now was between 175 and 200 pounds, and that it would be more realistic for him to shoot for a target weight range of 180 to 185, and try to hold steady in that zone. This would put him above the upper range of some weight charts for his age, frame, and height, but would be more realistic and achievable than his initial goal of 170.

Bob's desire to lose weight was based on both aesthetic (or vanity) and health concerns. Fortunately, there is a "tipping point" in the relationship between weight and health, where a small weight loss (or gain) can have a large effect on health status. This is good news for people trying to lose enough weight to prevent or reverse a particular health problem.

A decision to lose or maintain weight for *specific* health reasons should be based on clear data, such as one's blood pressure, lipid profile, glucose tolerance (type 2 diabetes mellitus and pre-diabetes), musculoskeletal problems (such as functional limitations from osteoarthritis), respiratory problems (including obstructive sleep apnea and obesity hypoventilation syndrome), and any other weight-related health indicators. Progress toward a health goal can be monitored by keeping track of the relevant health indicator (e.g., blood pressure, fasting glucose, lipids).

Setting a weight range goal will work best when tied to specific outcomes the person strongly desires, and these may or may not be health related. If the desired range is based on fashion trends or to avoid the stigma (significant in our culture) of being overweight, then those reasons should be carefully considered as to whether they are truly worth the effort. Young women in our (U.S.A.) culture feel pressure to become *too* thin, and malnutrition is a risk (especially for adolescent girls).

There are various weight tables and formulas you can use as guides for determining what weight you want to shoot for (such as the one Bob used), and these may or may not be relevant to your specific situation. Overall, studies show that very few people are able to lose more than 15% of their original weight and keep it off. Although research is limited in this area, 13% to 22% of overweight people in weight loss treatment programs maintain a weight loss of at least 10 pounds five years after the treatment. In a random sample of the general U.S. population, 14% reported maintaining an intentional weight loss of at least 10% of their original weight after one year.[1]

In her book *The Beck Diet Solution*, Judith Beck encourages her Cognitive Therapy clients to discover their "lowest maintenance weight"[2] by adhering to a strict weight loss program followed by an equally strict weight maintenance program. She asserts that there is a two pound margin of error surrounding the target weight and if you gain three pounds over the target you would have to work harder to regain control or risk an escalating weight problem (which would eventually take you back to your original weight, or more).

Large population studies that span many countries, cultures, and time frames, teach us that as societies become healthier (e.g., in terms of chronic disease and death rates), both average height and weight increase at about the same rate. In fact, the numbers reveal that people who are unusually fat or unusually thin have the poorest health. The surprise is that the healthiest people are the ones who are slightly overweight according to standard weight tables.[3]

Research findings also teach us that rapid weight loss, e.g., losing 25 pounds in six months, triggers powerful mechanisms in the brain and body to send signals that we are starving. This results in an outpouring of brain chemicals that trigger strong cravings for food, in some cases irresistible. So, losing no more than one to two pounds per month works best.

Perhaps your goal is simply to drop a few pounds from your present weight, or even to just stop gaining weight, both of which are fine goals to start with. Preventing weight gain is more important than losing weight, at least at first. It is much harder to lose excess weight than to keep it off in the first place, and even harder to maintain the weight loss. If you can prevent gaining five pounds a year, that amounts to fifty pounds you have kept off over ten years – a very significant achievement!

Chapter 3

Step 3: Learn about "willpower" and self-change

"Dieters do have willpower. Most dieters have lost weight before. They've just gained it all back, so their willpower is a little bit inconsistent."

– Judith Beck, Ph.D.[1]

"Patience and perseverance have a magical effect before which difficulties disappear and obstacles vanish."

– John Quincy Adams

WHAT YOU NEED TO KNOW

There is no question that how we think and make decisions affects our behavior in significant ways. Fortunately, we have learned much about how our "higher brain functions" can override our impulses and emotion-based behavior, if we so choose. Some people find self-control easier than others, but there are concepts and techniques that make it much more likely for us to stick to a plan, especially after it becomes routine. Willpower (in its modern and non-judgmental form), reframing, and being aware of the stages of self-change are all useful tools in our journey toward self-improvement.

MORE DETAILS

Willpower – what does it mean, and do we have any?

Most psychiatrists, addiction counselors and diet gurus avoid using the term willpower, believing it damages self-esteem, makes people blame themselves, or seems socially wrong or outdated. Many prefer the term "motivation" which, to me, implies the energy to make a choice and initiate an action can come from forces beyond our own control, either from unconscious drives inside us or from external sources. I have chosen to use the term "willpower" in this book because it is less ambiguous and says clearly that the impetus comes from one's free will, and is powerful.

While it is beyond the scope of this book to discuss the many meanings over time of the terms "free will" and "intentionality," and whether human beings actually possess any, I believe we are able to exercise freedom of choice and, in varying degrees, make unique decisions and valid commitments. Neuroimaging studies ("functional MRIs" which show brain activity as we perform tasks) demonstrate that conscious decision-making accounts for from twenty to fifty percent of brain activity, depending on the novelty and complexity of the task. Many of our everyday decisions are made in the pre-conscious mind – outside our immediate awareness, but readily brought into awareness. Thus, *our willpower* (also referred to as *conscious volition, intentionality*, or *self-control*) is a force we can call upon when necessary, and with some degree of freedom.

Of course, there is nothing new about advocating willpower as part of a plan to control weight and live a healthy lifestyle. The Reverend Sylvester Graham (1794 – 1851), for whom the Graham Cracker was named, promoted the idea that willpower and self-denial combined with a healthy diet (organic fruits, vegetables, whole grains) and exercise would eliminate "gluttony and obesity." He wrote, "The whole system of governing the head by the stomach instead of governing the stomach by the head is utterly wrong. Make your stomach the healthful minister of the body, and not the whole body the mere locomotive appendage of your stomach. Treat your stomach like a well governed child;

carefully find out what is best for it ... and then teach it to conform to your regimen." Needless to say Grahamism, which opposed alcohol, sex and celebrations, did not become popular.[2]

Graham approached willpower from an authoritarian and judgmental direction, and drastically overstated his case. Unfortunately, this kind of moralistic extremism is associated with "willpower" today, and tends to obscure the positive implications of the word. Self-denial, which became the main focus of Grahamism, is an entirely separate concept from willpower, and is not at all what I am proposing. In fact, when people confuse self-denial with willpower, they doom themselves to failure. Very few of us would stick to a plan which consistently required self-denial, and the feeling of being denied or deprived is why many people quit diets and other "health programs." The section on "reframing," toward the end of this chapter, will address ways to avoid thinking in terms of self-denial.

How to get the most out of your willpower

When people hear the term "willpower," many envision Sisyphus, from Greek mythology, who was condemned to repeat forever the same meaningless task of pushing a rock up a mountain, only to see it roll down again. That is because we usually only pay attention to our own willpower when we are having problems applying it to a difficult task. The majority of the time we use it without even being aware of it, such as when we decide to watch TV instead of reading, or vice versa. In the following sections, I will suggest ways to make willpower more accessible in order to increase your effectiveness in getting what you really want out of life.

Enhancing "won't power" and willpower

While we have little control over many aspects of our lives, our willpower gives us the powerful ability to control our own thinking and, to a large degree, our mindset. In this section, I will briefly summarize several lines of research that show how important this ability is, and that suggest ways we can enhance our willpower.

Walter Mischel, a well-know Professor of Psychology at Columbia University, conducted now classic studies of self-control and the delay of gratification. He showed that four-year-olds who were able to wait before taking a marshmallow offered to them (when asked to do so by an adult who promised a greater reward if they waited) had better outcomes later in life (such as better educational achievement and social competence) than four-year-olds who gobbled the first marshmallow offered. The longer the child was able to wait (delay gratification), the better the eventual outcome. Others have confirmed similar findings, showing that people who are able to exercise self-control (or willpower) do better in the long run than those who quickly succumb to temptation.

The part of the brain that makes humans unique, because of its size and complexity, is the cerebral cortex, and the part of the cortex that seems to be the seat of most of our self-control, judgment, and "rational" thinking, is the *prefrontal cortex*. Sophisticated neuroimaging studies have demonstrated regulatory pathways between the prefrontal cortex and the "lower" brain areas and systems that are responsible for hunger and craving. Such studies provide at least indirect evidence that willpower is a highly developed and integral part of the human brain, and that there are neural pathways which we use to inhibit self-defeating impulses.

Other research has confirmed that the pre-frontal cortex becomes activated whenever we *prevent* ourselves from doing something impulsive. This has been labeled by some as "won't power" (or "free won't") and the implication is clear: willpower is not simply a philosophical or fuzzy psychological notion; our brains are "wired" to be capable of resisting temptation and delaying gratification, if we work at it.

Psychological studies by Dr. Roy Baumeister showed willpower can be increased by step-wise exercise, using such techniques as holding your breath, standing on one leg, writing with your left hand (if you're right-handed), and skipping a meal. He also demonstrated experimentally that people can get tired of exerting their willpower and need rest before it can build up again. Other studies have confirmed that willpower is like a muscle to the extent that it becomes stronger when we exercise it, and is also subject to fatigue when we over-use it. When fatigued, willpower can recover with rest, just like a muscle.

And willpower can be budgeted, like any other limited resource. For example, if you need extra willpower to limit your eating and drinking at a party, do not do other things that day that require willpower (such as washing the car or window-shopping). The best news is that the more we use our willpower over time, the more of it we will have![3]

Martin Seligman, a psychologist at University of Pennsylvania, observed that there are two types of ways that people deal with frustration in the battle over their willpower. When a setback occurs, *optimists* say, "It was the situation. And that situation was unique. Anyway, it'll be different next time," or something to that effect. *Pessimists* are more likely to give up and blame themselves for the setback, also refusing to give themselves credit when progress is made.

Seligman used the term "learned helplessness" in describing the giving-up phenomenon, and emphasized that the opposite could be learned too, that is, to be more optimistic and to activate willpower. When an optimistic person makes a mistake, the attitude is, "It was a good learning experience." Unlike pessimists, optimists are quick to give themselves credit when they do something well. Teaching people to think more constructively is sometimes successfully used in the treatment of depression, which itself can include learned helplessness behavior and attitudes.[3]

Realistic optimism is very different from *false hope*. For example, it is not unusual for people to go on many diets throughout their life, repeatedly losing weight and then regaining it, deluding themselves into hoping "this time it will work!" After an initial period while the pounds are coming off easily and they feel wonderful (usually lasting about six months), their weight plateaus and they become disillusioned and lose their will to continue with the diet. The cycle repeats itself over and over, and with each new diet the person thinks, "I am ready now; this time I will stick to it!"

Many people who experience this roller-coaster pattern adapt to it and accept it, grudgingly, as a way of life, clinging to the false hope that "next time it will be different." False hope, for some, eventually leads to burnout, discouragement, giving up, and learned helplessness. Though common, the "false hope" way of thinking is not at all the same as the positive mindset I am talking about.

One popular definition of insanity is doing the same thing over and over and expecting different results! Hopefully, reading this book will show you some new ways to do things, so that even small changes in your behavior might have a large effect on your long-term health and happiness.

"Can't," "Won't," "Try," and "Will"

A common psychotherapy exercise in experiential psychology (e.g., Gestalt Therapy) is to teach people to substitute the words "I won't" when they start to say "I can't." The exercise is a very powerful illustration of taking full responsibility for your behavior. Do it yourself and you will see how potent the words we use can be, even in silent thought. Once you get in the habit of saying "I won't," it is not a difficult transition to learn to say "I will!" and mean it. Thus, the existence of willpower is affirmed.

As an example, consider the statement "I can't control my eating." Notice how the meaning shifts if I say, instead, "I won't control my eating." If I *won't* control it, then it is also possible that I *will* control it, if I so decide.

Of course, there are many things we truly can't do, but too often we think we can't do something we really might be able to do. The purpose of this simple exercise is to demonstrate the power of taking responsibility for your behavior.

A related exercise is to hold a ball in your hand. Another person nearby gives you the order "try to throw that ball!" First, you are paralyzed with indecision, until it dawns on you that you cannot "try" to throw something; you either do or do not. Most people then throw the ball and laugh in recognition of how much language can affect behavior. We use words like "try" and "can't" to avoid the responsibility of actually having to commit to action. We therefore learn to be less, rather than more, powerful.

Freedom and responsibility

There is a dilemma connected with the concepts of free will and freedom of choice, which is that with freedom comes responsibility, and that can make life seem more demanding. Drifting along in life, going with the flow, one seldom has to account for where one is or where one is headed. Taking full responsibility for one's own thoughts, actions, and even feelings is a key part of self-actualization and personal growth, but may not be for everybody.

Exercising willpower – using conscious volition – is something we do when necessary. Much of the time, though, we are in a more relaxed almost automatic mode of being. A popular saying in AA is "easy does it!" Trying too hard can be tiresome and self-defeating, and basking in the flow of life is a wonderful concept. What we really need is *balance* in our lives between play and work, freedom and responsibility. We thrive when we achieve the right balance between ease and struggle.

We humans gravitate toward shortcuts in our interactions with our environment (in order to avoid being overwhelmed by the thousands of decisions we might otherwise be faced with). We adopt social rules, prejudices, stereotypes, and superstitions to make decisions easier, and we often accept the dictates of an authority (whether familial, tribal, governmental, academic or religious) so we don't have to decide so much on our own. When a diet guru comes along, who might also be a respected authority figure, and gives us clear rules to follow that s/he guarantees will make us reach our desired weight, we tend to listen and hope s/he is right. That is why so many people try so many diets and drift from one food fad to another, none of which results in sustained healthy eating or significant long-term weight loss.

I have observed that even when people avoid responsibility for making difficult decisions, they often are quite resourceful when pursuing something they really want. A man who procrastinates for months about fixing the lawn mower and getting his yard in shape will waste no time buying a set of high performance golf clubs and arriving at the tee on time. A young woman who puts off cleaning and organizing her apartment for a year will immediately get to work helping a friend plan and organize a wedding. So, there is no inherent reason an overweight person, who has avoided serious weight management activities in the past, might not suddenly commit to making a sustained effort to adopt a healthier lifestyle – after reading this book, for example.

The factors that cause most adults to gain weight in the first place, especially if they were not obese as children, are *partly* determined by behaviors over which we exert conscious control. Harvard researcher Jeff Flier sums up the dilemma: "The whole issue of appetite and weight regulation in humans ... is at the interface of free will and determinism."[4] The often quoted Alcoholics Anonymous slogan is applicable here: *"I strive for the serenity to accept the things I cannot change; the courage to change the things I can; and the wisdom to know the difference."*

Framing and reframing

How we conceptualize a situation or problem can be compared to how a frame interacts with a painting. The right picture frame can bring out the subtle colors and make the whole seem more beautiful than the sum of the parts, or it can detract from the painting and make it appear less attractive. If one frame doesn't work well with a particular painting, we can reframe it with another that works better for us. This metaphor can easily be applied to problems or issues in our lives, and we can choose to mentally frame, or reframe, a problem in whatever way makes it more manageable.

When we consciously look at a glass as half full rather than half empty, we are doing what many therapists teach their patients to do: using willpower to reframe, or change a negative way of looking at a problem into one with positive features. This does not mean we should automatically tell a person who just lost a loved one, "Be happy, s/he is in a better place!" Usually, reframing is most useful when applied to our own situation. It should be done intelligently and sensitively, and the rule of thumb here is to reframe in a positive way unless there is a good reason not to. That is, do not use reframing as a way of putting on rose-colored glasses in order to deny or distort reality. A successful reframe is both potentially true (factual, realistic) and positive. "Half full" and "half empty" are both true, but only one is positive.

How we frame a concept has a large effect on how we act in relation to it and, therefore, on the outcome. Thoughts can become self-fulfilling prophecies. For example, if I think, "I can't do this," such a thought will itself make it less likely for me to succeed, whereas "I *can* do this" will increase the likelihood of success (assuming there is a possibility I can do it). If I think "she won't trust me," I am likely to behave in a way that will make it less likely for her to trust me, whereas thinking "I am looking forward to talking with her" will more likely elicit a favorable result.

If you think, "healthy foods (fruits and vegetables, for example) are taste-less," you are unlikely to adopt healthier eating habits for a lifetime. If you reframe the concept of healthy foods to "healthy foods are good and good for me!" you will more likely enjoy eating them. We can definitely use our will-power to change the way we think about, and frame, important aspects of our lives. The results can be dramatic.

I have often heard people say, after munching on high calorie chips, dips, nuts and other "appetizers" (usually along with high calorie drinks) for hours, "let's go eat. This is not a *real* meal." That is a frame which is guaranteed to result in consuming way more calories than needed. Saying to oneself "I sure ate a lot – I don't want any more" would be a more healthful and ultimately more useful frame.

In her book *Rethinking Thin*, Gina Kolata describes a man (who is a subject in a diet study) having a very hard time losing weight. Ron talks about how dif-ficult it is to control his eating. The book describes Ron's dilemma: "He could not resist the urge [to eat ice cream]. The more he tried not to think about it or to tell himself that his goal was to be thin, the more he had to have it. Finally, of course, he went to the freezer and dished it out. 'The only thing I can come up with is that the reasons I want to lose weight – I want to feel better, to look slimmer, to look better – are not powerful enough.' [Ron said]."[5]

What is interesting about Ron, as Kolata further describes the situation, is not how hard it was for him to resist eating high calorie food, but how easy it was for him to resist it when he framed it differently than "trying to lose weight." Ron made a decision as an adult to keep kosher, and never had a problem resisting food that he believed was not kosher. Kolata: "It is a para-dox, he [Ron] says. He knows from his own experience that it is possible to refuse food, to be totally uninterested in it, for religious reasons. But not, he fears, for reasons of staying thin." Ron says, "If someone said, 'Peanuts aren't kosher,' I would never eat a peanut again. But if someone said, 'Peanuts make you fat,' that isn't enough ... It is one thing to know that a handful of peanuts is 190 calories. It is another thing not to eat it. I have this knowledge now. The question is, Do I choose to use it or not?"[6] The human mind indeed works in mysterious ways.

For me, framing weight management in terms of using willpower is empowering, in that it gives me maximum control over my own destiny. Some people find it more useful to frame the challenge in terms of fighting a disease or addiction, and there is nothing inherently wrong with that. Both of those frames (disease and addiction) come with the risk, however, of trying to use "cures," "treatments," or programs (like a pill, a crash diet, or a 12-step program) that are inappropriate and will, therefore, lead to failure. So, use such frames with caution and awareness of the potential pitfalls.

Substituting the phrase "I won't" for "I can't," as suggested earlier, is a reframe. A similar kind of reframe is to say "I want" instead of "I need" or "I should." Talking in terms of what we *should* do, rather than what we *want* to do, is setting ourselves up for failure and self-reproach. As we used to say in the 1970s, "Don't should on yourself!" Language is terribly important in therapy and in self-improvement. We can use our willpower to change the language of our thoughts.

Where adopting a healthy lifestyle is concerned, a useful reframe is to look at our long-term welfare as opposed to short-term desires. I may think, "I *want* to lie on the couch munching popcorn and watching TV after dinner," but I know that if I take a walk instead I will feel much better later and, since it advances my plan, feel a sense of accomplishment as well. My old habit would be to say to myself: "I really *should* take a walk (but I don't want to!)." The useful reframe here is "I really *want* to take a walk more than I want to lie on the couch!" The word "want" can apply to both short- and long-term wishes, so I am not lying to myself with this reframe.

Caroline Davis, Robert D. Levitan and others did research which suggests the ability to think in terms of one's long term welfare correlates with lower weight. The heavier people in their study showed a tendency to make choices that would give them immediate payoff at the expense of their eventual well being.[7] This is similar to the findings of the marshmallow study discussed earlier.

If you feel hungry an hour before dinner and think "I must have something to eat right away," a useful reframe might be "I am hungry, but want to wait so I will really enjoy my dinner in an hour; anticipation is a good thing!" This may work for you (as it does for me), but it may backfire if it results in eating more food when dinner finally is ready. For some people, a healthy snack before dinner, rather than letting anticipation build, results in fewer calories consumed.

Much has been written about the pros and cons of eating snacks or multiple small meals vs. sticking with three meals per day, but the ultimate test is whether the behavior and how you think about it helps you approach your goal. Always ask yourself when evaluating a difficult decision: "Will this get me what I want in the long run?"

Getting thoughts, feelings and behavior in alignment

Reframing is a skill taught in a form of therapy known as Cognitive Behavioral Therapy (CBT). Chapter 13 gives a lot more detail about this method, but many of the techniques, like reframing, can be self-taught and practiced without a therapist being involved. As a therapy, CBT has been shown to help people learn to cope with anxiety, depression, eating disorders, and many other problems. The basic philosophy involves learning to change your thinking, including automatic thinking usually outside your conscious awareness, in a more rational direction.

The theory, which has been validated through much research, includes the premise that changing your thoughts can ultimately lead to changes in your feelings and behavior, so that all three (thoughts, feelings, and behavior) are in *alignment*, or are congruent.[8] A variant of CBT focuses on changing behavior first, then thoughts, and finally feelings. Regardless of the order of change, the end result of *alignment* is the most important aspect.

The Self-Change Process

If you have read this far, and have weight loss (or weight maintenance) as a serious goal, chances are you are at least in the Contemplation Stage as described by James Prochaska, Carlo DiClemente, and John Norcross in a series of articles reporting on their research into how people make important changes in their behavior over time. Their "Stages of Change Model" applies very well to weight management and is especially useful because it predicts and confronts the extremely common problem of early success and later failure. The model covers a time period of many years, and also deals with the possibility of relapse.[9]
Briefly, the stages are:

- **Pre-contemplation**. This is the "ignorance is bliss" stage before one is aware change might be needed. One may be aware s/he is overweight, but tend to shrug it off as "genetic" and not think of it as something to actually control.

- **Contemplation**. This crucial stage may last for years and is characterized by ambivalence. One may think, "I really should lose weight," and may even read about it and try a few diets in a half-hearted way. Words people use when they are in this stage are "can't," "won't," "might," "maybe," "we'll see," "I'll try," and, finally, "I want." A thought, feeling, comment from another, or event may trigger movement toward taking action.

- **Preparation**. Here is where serious planning begins. There will be more focused education and consideration of many of the issues covered in this book. If special supplies (e.g., notebooks, pedometer) are needed, they will be acquired. Time and space in one's schedule/environment are arranged. People say, "I'm going to do this!"

- **Action**. Now the plan is implemented. This stage tends to last from three to six months.

- **Maintenance**. This is perhaps the most important stage, and the one most often ignored. It consists of a continued commitment to sustaining new behavior, and lasts for many years or a lifetime. Changes in one's environment and even relationships may be required, so that the positive new behaviors will be encouraged and supported.

- **Relapse**. Commonly, a person will relapse and resume pre-Action behavior at some point (or points). Relapse, also called "a slip," can provide valuable information about ways the plan needs modification. After a relapse, a person may need to go back to the contemplation or preparation stage, or, if no major change in plan is indicated, go right back to maintenance.

None of the stages is absolute in any way, and people spiral back and forth from one stage to another as needed. It is important to realize that the self-change stages apply to all sorts of decisions you are trying to implement, and therefore you may be in one stage regarding one decision (e.g., eating less) and another stage regarding any other decision (e.g., exercising more, or reducing family stress).

In my experience, teaching people the stages, and helping them assess where they are in the process at any given time, empowers them to keep on track with their decision. Knowing the stages also helps us have realistic expectations of ourselves and prevents us from falling into common traps, such as relaxing our effort after three to six months of "successful" behavior change. Understanding the stages, therefore, is an extremely important component of exercising willpower in controlling weight.

Mostly, we want to have control over our eating

All things considered, most of us cherish our ability to decide what to eat, and make quite a production out of scanning the environment for potential food, acquiring it, preparing it, sharing it, and talking about it. A multi-billion dollar industry makes sure we are exposed to many food-related choices, and constant marketing and advertising vies for our attention, acceptance, and, ultimately, consumption. So, even if we opt out of making decisions in some areas of our life, we usually enjoy making them where food is concerned.

We appear energized around food decisions, eagerly sharing with one another our latest restaurant find, where we found the best strawberries, and our favorite recipe for Mediterranean chicken. My point is that, while we often avoid making difficult choices, we also value our freedom to pursue things we really want, such as good food. Most "diets" restrict this freedom and remove much of the adventure and excitement we normally feel about eating. Yet, by learning a few skills and following a plan, we can have it all: successful weight management under our own control, *and* joyful eating.

Chapter 4

Step 4: Learn how to manage stress

WHAT YOU NEED TO KNOW

It is important to recognize the role of stress in our lives and to take charge of how we manage it, or else it will manage us. How we respond to acute and chronic stress may determine our success when it comes to weight control. Emotional or impulsive eating is the most common way people gain unwanted weight, and there are ways to recognize and control this problem. Having positive and supportive relationships is also important when we try to change stress-related behavior.

MORE DETAILS

Stress reduction

Many people who struggle with weight control describe lives filled with chronic stress. For all of us it is important to find sources of inspiration and relaxation – and stress reduction. In our hectic culture, shopping (often for food), watching television, eating, and going out to eat have replaced other more healthy ways to find pleasure, satisfaction, and meaning.

We often eat to compensate for stress and anxiety, and the subsequent weight gain adds to a vicious cycle of more stress and anxiety, and so on and on. In a potentially "revolutionary" article published in 2007 research scientists at Georgetown University showed that in mice and other animals *chronic stress combined with a high fat diet can cause weight gain greater than the amount expected from calorie intake.* The lead researcher, Dr. Zofia Zukowska, talked about the future implications for the treatment of human obesity saying, "It's not just the stress. It's the combination of stress and the high-fat, high-sugary rich diet that is the humongous combo. There is some kind of interaction going on."[1]

"Comfort" or emotional eating and bingeing

A major problem with weight management is so-called comfort food. These foods, often rich and calorie-laden, are associated with pleasant memories from childhood and home cooking, or some other past emotion. While eating these foods later in life gives immediate emotional relief from many kinds of unpleasant feelings, or simply evokes positive emotions during times of boredom, in the long run this habit causes more problems than it solves.

One research study of people watching a movie demonstrated how strongly mood affects how much we eat. Professor Brian Wansink and colleagues at Cornell University assigned research volunteers to watch one of two movies:

"After the movies were over and the tears were wiped away, those who had watched Love Story had eaten 36 percent more popcorn than those who had watched the upbeat Sweet Home Alabama," said Wansink, author of the recent book *Mindless Eating: Why We Eat More Than We Think.*[2] "Those watching Sweet Home Alabama ate popcorn and grapes, but they spent much more time popping grapes as they laughed through the movie than they did eating popcorn. Wansink suspects that happy people want to maintain or extend their moods in the short term, but consider the long term and so turn to comfort food with more nutritional value. People feeling sad or depressed, however, just want to 'jolt themselves out of the dumps' with a quick indulgent snack that tastes good and gives them an immediate 'bump of euphoria.'"[3]

As so often is the case, our language reinforces the problem. "Comfort food," because it may contribute to our long-term unhappiness and poor health, should sometimes be called "discomfort food." We are incredibly good at using language to disguise and rationalize our weaknesses!

I refer to a tendency to be driven by a habit of overeating, especially a self-defeating one, as a "weakness" not out of a sense of moral outrage nor as an indication of psychiatric disorder. Weakness is part of the human condition. Research which has looked for evidence of psychopathology or mental illness in people who overeat has not revealed any consistent pattern. So, as far as we know, overeating, even when driven by strong emotions and habits, is not evidence of mental illness.

The following case example is not about a psychiatric disorder, even though the person described was in psychotherapy:

Joe was in a terrible marriage. Every night before bed he would sit by himself and eat a pint of butter pecan ice-cream. In therapy he realized the connection between his stressful situation and his seemingly uncontrollable eating. When the therapist would remind him of this problem behavior, he would say he intended to keep doing it until the marriage was over. Sure enough, after he and his wife separated he stopped his nightly ice-cream binge. He lost 10 pounds the following year, and his comment to the therapist was, "I told you."

People do what they choose to do and often shift suddenly to the Action Stage when they are good and ready. Joe was very conscious of his overeating and had a plan to end it. It did not involve a special "diet" or any other gimmick. It was simply *his* plan. If he had been unaware of his eating behavior, as many people are at times, the problem would have been much harder to solve.

It is a good idea to avoid all eating that is done in an automatic, unconscious way. For example, eating while doing something else, or multi-tasking (even reading or watching TV), often leads to overeating. Plus, one misses the pleasure of eating when one is not paying attention to the food and is hardly even aware of the taste of each bite. If we make an effort to be consciously *mindful* of our eating, we will be much less likely to overeat, and we will enjoy the process of eating more.

There are times when "comfort food" is eaten intentionally as part of a reasonable weight management plan. No food should be off limits, even relatively "junk" food from a purely nutritional standpoint. The trick is to incorporate such foods into an overall plan, and to compensate for overeating by temporarily cutting back at another point. It is when "comfort" eating becomes frequent automatic behavior, or leads to binge eating, that it is a problem.

Stress management

Chronic stress, both physical and psychological, can increase our weight through emotional eating and can impair our ability to control impulses and think rationally. There are many books and articles about stress and stress reduction, so I will mention only a few of my favorite techniques that are underutilized.

First, learning how to be in silence is free, easy, and very important. Pay attention to background noise (such as the TV being on) and make time to just *be* in a silent environment. Try taking a walk without a music player attached to your ears.

Don't fill every moment with activity. People today even avoid going to the bathroom without reading something, text messaging, or doing a puzzle! We seem to fear quiet contemplation. Silence, aloneness and calmness allow us to take in who we are and where we are in life in a powerful and subtle way. Rhythmic deep breathing can enhance our relaxation and provide much needed oxygen to our brain. Practice it daily.

Mindfulness, a technique in which a person becomes intentionally and non-judgmentally aware of his or her thoughts and actions in the present moment, is a very important way to be more aware, and appreciative, of our experiences. It is also necessary to be mindful of our eating if we hope to eventually control it.

If we have some silence and mindfulness in our lives, listening to peaceful music at times can calm and inspire us. Loud, excited, sensational music can have the opposite effect. Reading, too, is an excellent pastime, and quality reading can add much to our quality of life.

Being in the presence of nature and other forms of beauty is nourishing to our soul. Walk in a garden, zoo, art museum, by a river, or just sit and watch the birds. We overlook these important sources of inspiration that our species has benefited from for millennia, but that today's fast-paced society devalues.

One can practice Yoga, meditation, and other relaxation methods that might reduce stress and take her/his mind off eating. Appropriate exercise itself, if not obsessive, can relieve stress and even combat depression, as well as help with weight control.

Sexuality is an important source of relaxation, stress relief, and communion with something and/or someone outside ourselves, and can help us stay focused on our goal of losing weight. Many sexual concerns go unaddressed in our hectic (and over-sexed) society, and an honest self-analysis will tell you if you need to improve this area of your life. It is well known in psychiatric circles that people sometimes overeat to compensate for a lack of satisfying sexual pleasure. And, there is some evidence that having regular sex can help with weight control!

Loving relationships

A powerful example of using willpower to achieve a long-term goal of having loving relationships is how we might respond to our own whiney feelings such as, "I want more love and attention!" A rational, though difficult, response would be to convert that self-defeating thought into an intention to *give* more love and attention. To do that takes willpower and goes against our most powerful wish in the here and now. But, if we heed our wiser inner voice, we will most likely get what we need and be much happier in the long run. We can exercise our willpower so that we create a win-win situation, where a win-lose, or even lose-lose, outcome might have occurred.

Chapter 5

Step 5: Guard against "willpower fatigue"

"Man is a rational animal who always loses his temper when called upon to act in accordance with the dictates of reason."

– Orson Wells

"Weight control is difficult. It takes sustained effort on making a lot of small changes that can last."

– Martin Binks, PhD[1]

WHAT YOU NEED TO KNOW

Change is difficult, and our brains, like our muscles, are subject to fatigue. In addition, there are many psychological traps we fall into when we try to change habitual behavior, and the most common of these are listed in this chapter. In general, the first step in avoiding such traps is recognizing, and admitting, they exist.

MORE DETAILS

Overcoming "willpower fatigue" and resistance to change

At this point in your reading, you may be feeling tired, even discouraged, because you have read this far in books before and not even finished. You might be thinking, "Why should I invest time and energy in doing what this guy says? What does he know?"

This response is a normal reaction in the stage of Contemplation (as described in Step 3) and should be acknowledged. Now is a good time to do a self-analysis concerning possible causes of resistance to change. In psychiatry, specifically in psychodynamic psychotherapy, *resistance* to change is always expected, and one learns to "analyze the resistance first." For the purpose of this self-help book, that implies you are doing some degree of self-analysis, which I strongly encourage. So, now is the time to look inward, honestly and calmly, in order to understand why you may resist following through with the changes you say you want to make.

"I need a break"

Whether stated out loud, or expressed through behavior, this is the most common reason for people going off diets or abandoning a healthy lifestyle (e.g., moving from the Action stage back to Contemplation). You may be tired of changing your behavior, and strongly desire "time off" or "time out" from your constant self-improvement program.

Willpower fatigue, also known as self-control failure, has three major causes, according to Florida State University Professor of psychology Roy Baumeister. First, conflicting goals and standards undermine control, such as when the goal of *feeling better immediately* conflicts with the goal of eating less in order to *feel better in the long run*. Second, failure to keep track of (monitor) one's own behavior renders control difficult. Third, self-control depends on a resource that operates like strength or energy, and depletion of this resource makes self-control less effective. Having to make a lot of decisions ("decision fatigue"), even minor ones, has been shown to deplete self-control.[2]

One practical implication of this research is that you should expect, and be on guard for, lower willpower on days when you have made a lot of decisions. Another implication is to avoid the stress of having to make too many decisions by simplifying and structuring your weight management plan so that you can do what you have decided to do as part of a routine; make it a habit.

As discussed in Chapter 3, willpower can be budgeted and can be increased by using it regularly. The more we "exercise" it, the more of it we have!

It is important to recognize willpower fatigue and to give your mind a rest, but also important to overcome a pattern of frequently taking time off, which can effectively sabotage your goal of weight control. Lower your expectations for a while, if needed, but remember it is much harder to remove newly added weight than to prevent its acquisition in the first place. Weigh yourself at least every month so you don't get blindsided with an extra five pounds to work off!

Demoralization

This is very common, and may be another form of willpower fatigue, but deserves special mention. Many people feel demoralized after being repeatedly discouraged, and serial dieters certainly are in this group. What is needed is a pep talk, from someone on TV, from a book, from a friend, or from yourself. As in political rallies, phrases like "Yes I can!" shouted with enthusiasm and conviction give us a boost. If you are in a group support setting, the phrase becomes some variant of "Yes *we* can!" Entire communities have come together with a common goal of losing weight (for example, Oklahoma City; see www.thiscityisgoingonadiet.com).

Too much going on!

Psychologist Abraham Maslow developed a theory in the 1940s that is still useful today. He believed that we all try to satisfy our needs, but that we must satisfy basic ones before we can put much energy into ones that are on the "personal growth" end of a continuum. He conceptualized a pyramid, which he called the "hierarchy of needs," where fundamental needs (such as for air, food, water, and security) are at the base, and higher needs (such as relationships and seeking meaning) are at the top. For example, a person concerned with getting food and shelter is not in a position to work on improving his education.

The details of the theory are not as important as the general conclusion that we only have so much energy, and if a basic need is not being met, we are unlikely to pursue a less essential goal until the basic one is satisfied. A related concept is, "You cannot teach someone to play table tennis in a hurricane." So, you may initially fail to follow your weight management plan because you have other, higher priority, issues to deal with that are either extremely distracting or take up most of your energy. Come back to your weight management plan once things settle down. If your life seems to be in "chronic crisis," though, and things never settle down, you may need to get professional help.

Fear of failure

A very common factor in resistance to change is fear, and fear of failure is on the top of the list. Most people who struggle with weight control have tried diets only to see the weight come back with a vengeance. Repeated failure leads to feelings of helplessness and/or low self esteem. This book is written with the goal of greatly reducing your chances of failing. But there are no guarantees.

Fear of failure creates a mindset of "You can't fire me – I quit!" Many people give up on a difficult project in order to avoid the imagined shame, blame and guilt if they should fail in spite of their best efforts. The obvious problem with this is that quitting guarantees failure, while forging ahead at least keeps open the possibility of success. Success can include learning valuable lessons, feeling pride in persevering, and knowing that you did not quit.

Remember, failure in the short run does not guarantee failure in the long run, and progress does not follow a steady path. People who believe they have failed are often too hard on themselves and not giving themselves enough credit for honest effort and enduring commitment. When you feel discouraged or fear failure, use that as a signal to re-commit and to persevere. Learn from mistakes ("negative" experiences can provide the most valuable of all lessons). If you decide weight control through self-empowerment is not for you, that is your right and your decision. All I ask is that you read this book so that you have a very clear idea of exactly why this approach is not for you. The information you gain about yourself may well help you in other areas of your life and in any future attempts to control your weight.

Fear of success

Fear of the consequences of being thinner or healthier may also play a role in resistance. How will a "new you" fit in with the longstanding expectations of friends and family? What new expectations will be thrust upon you? Everyone knows that a person who can get things done is the first to be called on to do even more. So, in a way, fear of success can be as daunting as fear of failure.

Anger

Anger can play a role in resistance. Is your "inability" to lose weight really a passive-aggressive way to get back at, or control, someone else? Do you habitually take anger at others out on yourself? Be totally honest in your self-appraisal. With insight, anger can be channeled into energy to get done what you want. Acknowledge it, and change it from a negative to a positive.

Impatience

Another major source of resistance is impatience. Healthy and rational weight loss is a slow process, ideally involving losing on average one to two pounds per month until one's target weight range is reached. Then, continued, or increased, effort is required to maintain. Remember the target is not set in stone, and one can always slow down and expect less without loss of face. For some, a reasonable goal would be to not gain weight this year. This slowness can be frustrating for some people – you know who you are. The only answer to this problem is to realize that slow and steady wins the race, acknowledge your frustration, and cope with it.

"My body has become my enemy!"

A similar kind of frustration occurs as we age and our body changes. There comes a point when the way we have eaten all our adult life suddenly turns on us and adds pounds. Again, one must be aware that such physiological changes are a normal part of surviving into middle and old age, and, like so many other aspects of our life, require us to adapt.

Indecision

Early in my psychiatry residency training program, I learned this saying: "Not making a decision is making a decision." It was one of the most useful things I learned. Many people, when confronted with an internal conflict, become paralyzed with anxiety, indecision, and inaction. This often takes the form of avoidance or procrastination. But the inaction itself results in missed opportunities and allows the external situation to evolve without the person's input. The job goes to someone else, the spouse decides to leave, or the pounds keep piling on (if you can't decide to change your eating/exercising habits, for example). Indecision sometimes works to avoid the heavy feeling of responsibility and "decision-fatigue," but usually the problem gets worse the longer it is left alone. The solution, of course, is to use your willpower to make the best decision you can given the information available. Of course, in some situations the wisest decision might be to "do nothing."

Being "good" or "bad"

As children, most of us looked up to our parents (or parent figures) and tried to please them, and at other times we were determined to say "no" and do the opposite of what they wanted. As adults, we still have a tendency at times to conform ("be an angel") and at other times to rebel ("I don't know what got into me!"). We each have a childlike part of our self that wants what it wants when it wants it, and a parent-like part that tells us what is best for us. Somewhere in the middle is a rational component that mediates between the two extremes. This is where the kind of willpower I am concerned with is lodged.

Many people struggling with weight management issues play the "good child" conformist role at times, and the "bad child" rebel role at other times. So it goes with the diet yo-yo: "I'm being good this week, nothing but salads" or "I was bad last week, I ate cheeseburgers and fried chicken." "Tomorrow I'm going to get on the good foot." Our rational self asks, "What is best for the long run; what will make me happy? Do I really want to stay on this roller-coaster?" Use your willpower to harness the rebellious energy you still have (and should cherish) and apply this energy to your commitment to stay on track with your plan.

All-or-none thinking and perfectionism

Another kind of roller-coaster is all-or-none thinking. When we are following a plan, we want to do it all the way. When we get frustrated, we want to chuck the whole thing. Perfectionism is a form of all-or-none thinking. Just remember the old saying, "The perfect is the enemy of the good," and do the best you can in the moment. Overachieving leads to burnout. If you find you are forcing yourself to get it all right, maybe you need to slow down and let your brain absorb and adjust for a while. Don't be afraid to lower your goal (e.g., from losing weight to not gaining) if you need to. But do so thoughtfully, not impulsively.

Rigidity

This is related to perfectionism, but slightly different. Carrying out a plan successfully requires flexibility; both the ability to hold steady, and also to roll with the punches. Relapse, for example, can teach us to modify our plan if it was too ambitious. Sticking to a plan just because we said we would, and rigidly refusing to change course or make adjustments, is a form of self-sabotage. Following unreasonable rules just because "that's the way it's always done" or "everybody knows that!" can be problematic. We need to be able to shift gears – to "think outside the box" when creativity is called for, and "think inside the box" when we want to benefit from the experience of others (and not reinvent the wheel).

Being overly optimistic or pessimistic

Habitually thinking, "This will be a cakewalk! No problem!" can set you up for disappointment, just as thinking, "This is way too hard. I'll never do it, so why bother" can set you up for certain failure. The trick is to be both up-beat and realistic.

"I deserve a reward!"

If you have been successfully working on changing your eating and exercise patterns for some time, you will encounter situations where someone will say to you "This is a special occasion, so go ahead and eat that cake!" The cake is not the issue, but the implication behind the statement is. People observing your healthier lifestyle will assume you are in a constant state of self-deprivation, and will want to see you "loosen up." It is important to them to feel okay about their own "indulgences." The problem with your buying into that theory is that it discounts the fact that you already are eating (and exercising) the way you want to. You are not depriving yourself – in fact, by doing what you want, you are indulging yourself. Your ongoing healthy lifestyle is its own reward.

Another problem with going back to old unhealthy habits, even temporarily, is that such "special occasions" come up frequently: out-of-town trips, weddings, graduations, birthdays, holidays, cruises, office parties, etc. etc. Add the special occasions with their special "indulgences" or "rewards" up over the course of a year and you have put on an unwanted five to ten pounds.

Temptation to go back to your old ways will fade over time, and you will be amazed with yourself when you are enjoying a trip to New York, eating very well, and still sticking to your plan. Special occasions are even more special when they don't throw you off your chosen path.

"I have accepted my body the way it is"

Perhaps you are overweight, obese even, but it isn't that big a deal to you. You feel constant social pressure to change, however, and know that you are stigmatized by some as "fat" and presumably "undisciplined." Maybe you have a bit of hypertension controlled by medication, or a knee that bothers you at times, but you feel these are not big deals, either. Some overweight people live long, happy lives, and you can think of several examples. Why should you struggle with your eating which is a very important source of socialization and pleasure for you?

Well, maybe you shouldn't. Many people who embark on difficult programs to change their lifestyle are not really doing it for themselves, but because of external pressure. If you are happy and reasonably healthy, and don't mind being large, then perhaps no weight management plan will make sense. Before deciding to give up on weight management, though, review the personal reasons why you chose this goal in the first place (Step 1). Remember, adopting a healthy lifestyle of eating less (especially "junk" food) and exercising more has benefits that are independent of weight loss. The choice is yours.

Get help if you need to, but keep on going

If you really do want to control your weight and/or have a healthier lifestyle, and continue to experience significant fatigue or resistance as described in this chapter, consider getting help from a counselor or therapist. You might have to do some research plus trial and error to find a good fit between you and a therapist.

Knowledge is power, and self-knowledge is no exception. The solution to overcoming willpower fatigue and resistance to change is acknowledging its presence and resolving to stay on track. Self-sabotage is common, but unnecessary. Don't let it get the best of you. Keep on reading this book! Do the **easy action steps** in Chapter 11!

Chapter 6

Step 6: Learn the basics about diet and exercise

WHAT YOU NEED TO KNOW

The basic principles of sensible eating and exercising are very simple, and were summarized by a prominent nutrition professor writing in 2007:

"Basic dietary principles are not in dispute: eat less; move more; eat fruits, vegetables and whole grains; and avoid too much junk food. 'Eat less' means consume fewer calories, which translates into eating smaller portions and steering clear of frequent between-meal snacks. 'Move more' refers to the need to balance calorie intake with physical activity. Eating fruits, vegetables and whole grains provides nutrients unavailable from other foods. Avoiding junk food means to shun 'foods of minimal nutritional value'—highly processed sweets and snacks laden with salt, sugars and artificial additives. Soft drinks are the prototypical junk food; they contain sweeteners but few or no nutrients. If you follow these precepts, other aspects of the diet matter much less. Ironically, this advice has not changed in years."[1]

I would only add that a little exercise goes a long way toward improving health, that incorporating "spontaneous exercise" and "non-exercise activity" into our lives is important, and that exercise alone, without dietary changes, is usually not sufficient for weight control (although the relative importance of exercise varies greatly among individuals). Also, fad diets and diet gimmicks are often useless in the long run and may do more harm than good. Finally, diet drugs have very limited value, if any, and do not work in the absence of lifestyle change. Surgery for weight reduction should be used only when clearly medically indicated.

MORE DETAILS

One can lose weight by severely restricting one's intake or cutting down on the variety of food one enjoys, but such methods often interfere with optimum nutrition and quality of life. Also, one can lose weight without exercising and becoming more fit, but that, too, would be a less healthy choice. We should remember that, in general, we eat for many reasons – pleasure, tradition, culture, energy, social, political, religious, philosophical – and that food is not medicine. Today, there are so many health claims and counterclaims about the value of one type of food over another that we can easily be confused and overwhelmed. In his book *In Defense of Food,*[2] Michael Pollan argues that "nutritionism" is an embryonic science and offers little, if any, worthwhile guidance. For example, we were told by such "scientists" that we should be eating more beta carotene, leading to many people taking "antioxidant" supplements, which we now know may do more harm than good (research shows that taking beta carotene and/or vitamins A and E, unless there is a deficiency, does no good and may do harm; taking iron supplements can also be harmful, unless medically indicated). Rather than focusing on the latest supplement fad, according to Pollan, we should do what our ancestors did, and simply eat a variety of foods provided by nature, not factories.

Healthy food choices

Fortunately, we do have the ability to choose a variety of satisfying and healthy foods (except for relatively unusual examples of food allergies or intolerances). While long lists of "good" and "bad" foods are cumbersome and faddish, some general guidelines about food can be helpful. There are food categories that we can eat more of that give us a better deal when we want to lose weight. For example, "low energy density" foods with a high moisture content (many soups, salads, most vegetables, fresh fruits) are more filling and have fewer calories per bite than their calorie-dense counterparts (butter, bacon, fried foods, cookies, creamy dressings and sauces, etc.). Also, foods high in simple sugar (glucose, sucrose, high fructose corn syrup) tend to create a rebound phenomenon where the more we eat, the more we crave. This is because the rapidly changing glucose level in the bloodstream affects hunger receptors in the brain, and because of insulin induction. Sugary drinks (soft drinks, Gatorade, fruit juices) should be avoided (except perhaps for the "diet" forms that contain sugar substitutes).

There has been much written and debated about "good" and "bad" carbohydrates (the so-called glycemic index), and about whether carbohydrates are the biggest culprit when it comes to unwanted weight gain. There are no final answers. Carbohydrates (carbs) are everywhere in our food preferences, so the best general rule is to limit sugars in the diet and generally eat carbs in moderation and eat them along with other foods that slow down glucose absorption (such as lean proteins, healthy fats, and high-fiber fruits, vegetables and grains). Many nutritionists advise people to avoid *white* carbohydrates such as sugar, white breads, and plain rice or pasta (brown rice and whole grain bread and pasta are preferred).

Moderation, in fact, is the overriding rule in striving for a healthy lifestyle.

We should eat less saturated fat (fat that is solid at room temperature) and relatively more of the kind that comes in liquid form (like olive or canola oil). Recent evidence has shown that trans-fats are harmful to our cardiovascular system and should be avoided. Fortunately, food labeling now makes that easier. Fats in general have high energy density and have more calories per unit of weight than protein and carbohydrates. Some studies conclude that fats provide less of a feeling of fullness or satiety than other food types, but others contend the opposite. Whether a particular food helps us feel satisfied and thus leads to less calorie consumption seems to be highly variable from person to person. Many people who are able to maintain their target weight range over a long period of time limit their fat intake to low-moderate levels (24% of total calories).[3] Others claim that limiting carbs is the key factor.

Protein is a very important part of our diet and we should get most of it from sources which are relatively low in saturated fat and high in beneficial nutrients (fish, lean meat, low-fat milk and cheese, eggs, nuts, beans). Some experts claim that protein also makes you feel full longer than do fats and carbs. Production of meat on a large scale is unhealthy for the planet, in terms of efficiency of energy use and production of greenhouse gasses. So, as mentioned earlier, food choice involves much more than deciding what is more or less healthy for individuals.

Drinking lots of water helps some people avoid reaching for calorie-laden drinks or snacks, and helps them feel full. Studies of using water as part of a weight-loss program have been inconclusive, however. It is possible to drink too much water and suffer from water intoxication, which can be fatal.

Chewing sugarless gum and using long lasting sugar-free candies helps some people avoid eating when they feel like putting something in their mouth. Chewing thoroughly and taking more time to eat can be helpful and allow your brain time to get the signal from your gastrointestinal system that you are full. Brushing your teeth after eating can be a marker that you are finished until the next meal, and is a good idea anyway.

Food labels now contain useful information, and healthy eating requires familiarity with the labeling format. With a little practice, it does not take long to quickly scan a label for key information, such as serving size (very important), calories, protein, types of fat, fiber, sugar, and sodium. The ingredient section lists food components in order; if sugar or corn syrup is number one or two on the list, think again about buying the product. Search on the Internet about "how to read a food label" for more information.

Research shows that our mood affects how we use food labels. In one study, popcorn was offered to two groups of volunteers, one group that had been told to read and write about themes that made them happy, and the other about sad themes. The groups were subdivided into those who were shown nutritional information about the popcorn, and those who weren't. The sad group dramatically cut down its intake when shown the information. The happy group was already eating less, so there was no change when they reviewed the same information.[4]

Portion size

Much research supports the fact that portion size is a major determinant of how much we eat. For example, Brian Wansink, Professor of Marketing and of Applied Economics at Cornell University, conducted several studies which showed that:

- Moviegoers ate 45% more popcorn when served in a large tub compared to a medium sized container.
- People watching a movie ate twice as much M&Ms from a large bag compared to a small bag.
- In neither of the above studies were the research subjects able to guess the number of calories they had consumed; people consistently underestimate the amount they eat.
- While people tend to acknowledge that portion size and container size may influence other people, they often wrongly believe they themselves are unaffected.[5]

We all suffer from "portion distortion" when we estimate the amount of food we consume, not only at mealtime, but when we snack and eat without being mindful (automatic eating). To see whether you have this problem, check out the Portion Distortion Quiz on the Internet (http://hp2010.nhlbihin.net/portion/).

For decades, American food and diet writers have discussed the "French paradox," noticing that people in France eat lots of high calorie meats, breads and dairy products, and yet tend to be thinner than people from the United States. Many theories have been offered to explain this paradox, and it seems that three factors are important: French people enjoy food, but in smaller amounts (smaller portions); the French traditionally spend more time eating (are more mindful); and they tend to walk and cycle more (more exercise). Unfortunately, as our fast-food culture spreads around the world, the "obesity epidemic" is also spreading to other countries, including France.

Americans are immersed in a mass-produced food culture that emphasizes "super size" portions and huge amounts of fat and sugar. Between 1967 and 2003 sugar consumption in the U.S. increased from 114 pounds to 142 pounds per person per year and has continued to rise to an estimated 170 pounds in 2006![6] A few years ago I toured an ice cream factory that exports its popular products all over the world. The guide said that the ice cream they sell in the U.S. market is loaded with extra fat and sugar compared with what they export. Clearly, the U.S. food environment is a major factor contributing to the startling increase in obesity (especially child obesity) in this country and now world wide.[7]

Official dietary guidelines for Americans (2005)

Another, more official, way to say some of what I have said above about healthy eating comes from the U.S Government. This information contains extra detail that can be helpful. I have extracted a few important passages from the lengthy science-based dietary guidelines for Americans (2005):[8]

- To maintain body weight in a healthy range, balance calories from foods and beverages with calories expended.
- To prevent gradual weight gain over time, make small decreases in food and beverage calories and increase physical activity.
- Some proposed calorie-lowering strategies include eating foods that are low in calories for a given measure of food (e.g., many kinds of vegetables and fruits and some soups). The healthiest way to reduce calorie intake is to reduce one's intake of added sugars, fats, and alcohol, which all provide calories but few or no essential nutrients.
- Lifestyle change in diet and physical activity is the best first choice for weight loss. A reduction in 500 calories or more per day is commonly needed. When it comes to body weight control, it is calories that count—not the proportions of fat, carbohydrates, and protein in the diet. However, when individuals are losing weight, they should follow a diet that is within the Acceptable Macronutrient Distribution Ranges (AMDR) for fat, carbohydrates, and protein, which are

- 20 to 35 percent of total calories [from fat],
- 45 to 65 percent of total calories [from carbs], and
- 10 to 35 percent of total calories [from protein].

- Diets that provide very low or very high amounts of protein, carbohydrates, or fat are likely to provide low amounts of some nutrients and are not advisable for long-term use.

- Choose a variety of fruits and vegetables each day. In particular, select from all five vegetable subgroups (dark green, orange, legumes, starchy vegetables, and other vegetables) several times a week.

- At least half the grains in your diet should come from whole grains.

- Consume three cups per day of fat-free or low-fat milk or equivalent milk products.

- Consume less than ten percent of calories from saturated fatty acids and less than 300 mg/day of cholesterol, and keep *trans*-fatty acid consumption as low as possible.

- [Most fats in your diet should come] from sources of polyunsaturated and monounsaturated fatty acids, such as fish, nuts, and vegetable oils.

- When selecting and preparing meat, poultry, dry beans, and milk or milk products, make choices that are lean, low-fat, or fat-free.

- Consume less than 2,300 mg (approximately 1 tsp. of salt) of sodium per day.

Other sources of nutritional and weight management information

There are several relatively unbiased and trustworthy publications available to the public, such as health letters put out by prestigious universities and clinics. *The Nutrition Action Health Letter*, published by Center for Science in the Public Interest, is one example. It not only summarizes the latest nutrition and health research, but also rates specific food products by name and gives pricing.

Consumer Reports is helpful as well. The June 2007 issue, for example, thoroughly covered and rated diet books and diet plans. Their conclusions:

None has shown long-term success, but the top two plans were *The Volumetrics Eating Plan* (Barbara Rolls, Ph.D.) and Weight Watchers. The article stressed that people tend not to stick with any of the reviewed diet plans, partly because they become bored with the restrictions. Some other useful conclusions from the article were:

- Don't skip breakfast.
- Watch the kind and amount of fat in your diet.
- Watch serving sizes.
- Increase activity.
- Fill up on low-density foods (soups, salads, fruits, vegetables).
- Weigh yourself regularly so you can head off weight gain early.

For many people, weighing regularly, for example once a month, is a good and easy way to monitor progress. You may also want to monitor blood pressure, lipids, and any other health indicators you are trying to change.

"Diets" don't work well

Diets have been with us for centuries. Over 2000 years ago, Hippocrates wrote about the virtues of eating less and exercising more. Calorie counting became a national obsession in the early part of the twentieth century after Irving Fisher and Eugene Fisk published the bestselling *How to Live – Rules for Healthful Living Based on Modern Science* (1915). They emphasized how people delude themselves when they think "many articles such as candy, fruit, nuts and peanuts, often eaten between meals, 'do not count,' [and when they] overlook accessories, such as butter and cream, which may contain more food value than the entire meal put together." They warned, "Nature counts every calorie very carefully. If the number of calories taken in exceeds the number used by the body, ... the excess accumulates in fat or tissue. ... If reduction in the amount of energy food and an increase in the amount of exercise is made, no power on earth can prevent a reduction in weight." The calorie-counting craze lasted for a decade before it was replaced with various other diet fads, many of which come into favor and go out of style repeatedly.[9]

The problem with the calorie-counting fad and all the others is not that they are illogical (some are, some aren't), but that they are swallowed whole by a gullible population that doesn't really understand the science behind the claims nor the basic principles of behavior change, as outlined in this book. Estimating calories consumed and expended, for example, can be helpful, but is not practical if taken to extremes and must be part of an overall approach to healthier living.

The research on diets, which is limited, generally shows that "diets" do not work well. More importantly, people dislike diets and rarely stay on them for more than a year. There are two basic kinds of diets: ones that set out an *eating plan*, with recipes and lists of "good" and "bad" foods (for example, Atkins, South Beach, Volumetrics, The Zone), and diets that involve *counting* points or calories.

My objection to diet books and diet plans that list foods to eat and foods to avoid, and often include recipes and "quick start" and time-limited "guaranteed" fast weight loss gimmicks, is that they are boring, based on poor science, and usually too complicated and/or too restrictive for most people to follow. Not many of us are willing to live under those conditions long-term.

When you say to yourself and others, "I am going on a diet starting tomorrow!" or, "I am going on the Movie-Star-of-the-Month-South-Mediterranean-high-fiber/low-sugar diet!," you are implying that a diet is something you go on, which also means it is something you go *off*. The concept of "diet" as it is commonly used today is that it is temporary and extraordinary. No wonder the research shows over and over that people do not stick with them.

Weight Watchers is in the category of *counting* (points, in this case), and usually also involves meeting in a group. Weight Watchers is less about deprivation than many diets, but also imposes hard-to-maintain conditions. For one thing, you must have a group of other Weight Watcher participants to meet with. Over time, people drop out for dozens of valid reasons, and usually shortly after the group stops meeting (and the regular weigh-ins stop) the eating behavior reverts to earlier, ineffective patterns. That is because the main power for the change came from outside the self, and never became an integral part of one's individual behavioral repertoire. (Groups of supportive people with similar goals can be very effective, though, as will be discussed in Step 8). The Weight Watchers point system, which some people use without the group component, can be helpful, but is more complicated than simple awareness of calories and healthy eating would be.

Although, in general, knowledge is power, too much information can be confusing and even paralyzing. The amount of press, Internet, and bookshelf space given to food-nutrition-lifestyle-health-exercise topics is astounding. As will be discussed in Step 7, any reasonable diet plan or counting method can work if it is something you can live with for a long period of time.

The best "diet" (using the older meaning "habitual nourishment") is a life-long pattern of following reasonable nutritional guidelines, but also contains the foods you like, in reasonable amounts and frequencies. The trick is how to change your eating preferences and lifestyle habits (including activity level) to match what is healthy and realistic for the rest of your life.

Exercise and "non-exercise activity"

An effective exercise plan requires some basic education, but need not be unpleasant. The most economical way to exercise, especially for people with crowded schedules, is to incorporate it into daily life. Some refer to this as "spontaneous exercise." For example, if you are sitting, lift your legs up and down for a while; stand on one leg while brushing your teeth; do isometric exercises throughout the day (search the Internet for examples of isometric exercises). If you have access to stairs, use them. For example, if I have been sitting for a long time and have stairs nearby, I will just go up and down a flight several times as a break from whatever I was doing.

The more sedentary we are, the higher our risk for obesity. Our modern lifestyles encourage sitting rather than moving: comfortable chairs and cars, video games, remote controls, riding mowers, etc. Research at the Mayo Clinic by James Levine, MD, has clearly shown that the more we move throughout the day, the more weight we lose (or don't gain). He calls this kind of movement NEAT, which stands for Non-Exercise Activity Thermogenesis. For most of us, NEAT accounts for far more of our daily calorie expenditure than formal exercise does (even fidgeting uses calories!). Levine found that thin people are on their feet an average of 2.5 more hours a day than their overweight counterparts.

NEAT is responsible for between 20 percent (in very sedentary "couch potatoes") and 50 percent of our total daily energy expenditure. Most of the rest of our energy expenditure is due to "basal metabolism" (calories used when we are at complete rest) which accounts for up to 60 percent; and "thermic effect of food" (digestion, absorption, storage) which accounts for 10 to 15 percent. Levine discovered that our individual NEAT level is largely biologically determined (possibly genetically) and that people with a naturally low level can be taught to increase their "non-exercise activity." He recommends that we aim for 40 percent NEAT by changing the way we work, such as standing while working and walking around during meetings and while on the phone. He uses a treadmill going very slowly (1 mph) throughout the day (a "walking workstation"); this kind of easy activity doubles our metabolic rate and uses an extra 100 calories per hour (compared to sitting). This would be a great way to watch TV![10]

We can all incorporate more walking into our lives. Walking to the store or restaurant instead of driving, and (if you drive) not parking too close to where you are going, are helpful. As little as twenty minutes of moderate walking (2 to 4 mph) several days per week has been shown to be beneficial for cardiovascular fitness. Slower walking may burn as many calories per hour for some (overweight) people as rapid walking, but may not have as much cardiovascular benefit.

Walking is a great way to get exercise, fresh air, a change of scenery and a break from work. It also provides an opportunity to think or just clear your mind. Several research studies have demonstrated that moderate aerobic exercise such as rapid walking has antidepressant and anti-anxiety effects, too. For example, Duke University researchers found that 30 minutes of brisk exercise three times a week was as effective as antidepressant medication in relieving symptoms of depression, and that patients who continued exercising had a lower relapse rate after ten months than patients taking medicine.[11]

For some, safety concerns or bad weather may prevent much walking to stores or in parking lots. Indoor walking – e.g., mall-walking – can be a good alternative. Even so, it makes sense to put in the effort to find pleasant and safe places to walk outdoors, and if your neighborhood doesn't have them, consider moving to a more walking-friendly area.

"Did he just say 'consider moving'?! Isn't that extreme?!," you may be thinking. But if you think about it, it is not so strange. We change locations all the time, and for a variety of reasons. Quality-of-life factors (like having access to sidewalks or biking paths) may not be quite as important as affordability and security, but they do enter into the equation. Personally, I enjoy walking so much that it influenced my choice of a region of the country in which to live and work (for the moderate climate) and has been a factor in where I chose to live within my current city each time I moved (6 moves in 25 years).

A very simple exercise, taught in some Yoga classes, is to tense your lower abdominal muscles throughout the day (imagine you are drawing your lower abdomen slightly in toward your backbone). Combined with good posture and "alignment," this will do a lot for your core muscles and won't take any extra time. This combination will also improve the way you look and you will actually be taller and thinner!

Learning to do Kegel exercises of the perineal (pelvic floor) muscles is important for a variety of reasons and can be done at any time – an excellent way to multitask!

Moderate aerobic exercise (walking, etc) has many health benefits, but it is important to put it in perspective. It should be done for pleasure and to feel well, not primarily to lose weight. For most of us, moderate exercise without dietary changes will not result in significant weight loss (although exercise is a key factor in *maintaining* weight once significant weight has been lost – see Step 7).

Not all exercise builds muscle mass, so try to include some form of progressive resistance strength training. Muscles use more energy even when we are at rest than fat does. The more muscle mass we have, the easier it will be to lose weight and keep it off. This is why men, who usually have a higher ratio of muscle to fat, have an easier time losing weight than women. Also, as we lose weight, we may lose muscle mass, so strength-building becomes even more important. Strength-building exercise can help prevent osteoporosis and, by strengthening our lower extremities, also prevent falls that can lead to serious injuries. Adding exercises that increase flexibility and balance also reduces our chance of injury. Be sure to do a warm-up routine before doing any exercise or stretching. Even people with severe physical limitations can learn exercises that will benefit them.

Physical activity recommendations from the dietary guidelines for Americans (2005):

- Engage in regular physical activity and reduce sedentary activities to promote health, psychological well-being, and a healthy body weight.
- To reduce the risk of chronic disease in adulthood: Engage in at least 30 minutes of moderate-intensity physical activity, above usual activity, at work or home on most days of the week.
- For most people, greater health benefits can be obtained by engaging in physical activity of more vigorous intensity or longer duration.
- To help manage body weight and prevent gradual, unhealthy body weight gain in adulthood: Engage in approximately 60 minutes of moderate- to vigorous-intensity activity on most days of the week while not exceeding caloric intake requirements.
- Achieve physical fitness by including cardiovascular conditioning, stretching exercises for flexibility, and resistance exercises or calisthenics for muscle strength and endurance.

Diet drugs

Stimulants of various kinds can reduce appetite, and some say smoking also can, so both are used as aids to weight loss. I oppose them because the health risks from the drug or tobacco product outweigh the supposed benefits to weight maintenance. Orlistat (Xenical, Alli) is FDA approved for the treatment of obesity and works by preventing dietary fat from being absorbed. It is difficult to take as prescribed (taken before meals which have a relatively low fat content), has only modest benefit, has significant gastrointestinal side effects, and is not a substitute for a healthy lifestyle.

Antidepressants and anti-anxiety drugs are sometimes prescribed to help people take better care of themselves, but these drugs can cause weight gain. If anxiety and/or depression are keeping you from concentrating on your health, seek treatment for those conditions. You may find that simply using the steps in this book will give sufficient relief so that you can get on with your weight management plan, but if more is needed, consult a therapist (who may or may not prescribe drugs or refer you to someone who will).

There may be some powerful new weight control drugs in the pipeline (such as canabinoid receptor blockers), but it seems that for now they are pipe dreams. When the big one passes the FDA and hits the market, I am sure you will hear a lot about it. In any case, you can be sure it will be expensive, have limitations, and may have serious known and unknown side effect.

The joy of eating and moving

Eating is one of the most pleasurable and sociable things we do. We can maximize our joy of eating by bringing it in harmony with our other joys, such as moving our bodies and living long lives with family and friends. There is every reason to assume that a healthy diet will also be a fun diet, including our favorite foods from the past and, importantly, new favorite foods we discover as we go. Healthy eating is an adventure made more and more enjoyable by the global marketplace and the ready access we now have to a wide variety of food from all over the world.

Variety in food may be the spice of life, but it is not a simple equation. Research suggests that overall variety in one's diet may correlate with a healthier diet, but too much variety at one meal (such as in a smorgasbord or buffet) leads to eating more. Also, the availability of a wide variety of tempting foods and snacks results in more calories consumed. I am encouraging variety and branching-out as a way to become familiar with different foods for the purpose of having more choices when it comes to planning healthy meals. Once healthy eating habits are established, however, there is some evidence that consistency of diet from day to day and week to week is helpful, as is a narrowing of variety within each food group (except fruits).

There is much evidence from research that food preferences are learned and culturally determined, so we can teach ourselves to like healthy foods as much, or more, than we liked less healthy foods. A good example is how people have trained their taste buds to prefer skim milk to whole milk, even though at first it seemed watery and not at all like the creamy milk they had grown up with. Once one adjusts to skim milk, whole milk seems much too thick and rich. Similarly, if you cut back on sugar for awhile, you might find you will think "Too sweet!" when you go back to the level of sweetness you had previously preferred.

Fortunately, popular demand for healthier food has resulted in more choices for consumers. Many supermarkets now feature locally grown, seasonal, organic, and other relatively healthy food choices, and some grocery stores specialize in healthier foods. Such stores are usually attractive, interesting, and staffed by friendly and knowledgeable people. And some restaurants have added menu items that are suitable for a health-conscious diet. Many people now are finding that eating in ways that are less harmful to the planet (e.g., by consuming less meat and fewer processed foods, and by supporting local small farms) gives them even more satisfaction than simply "eating healthy" does.

Variety is a positive development where exercise is concerned. No more does "exercise" require regimented calisthenics or brutal sessions on workout machines (unless you enjoy these forms). Biking, hiking, dancing, playing – all are ways to enhance our enjoyment of the moment and our relationships with others.

Being healthy is fun in and of itself, and the process of becoming and staying healthy is also enjoyable. Remember, the glass of life is half full, not half empty!

Chapter 7

Step 7: Learn from others' experience

WHAT YOU NEED TO KNOW

There are thousands of accounts of people who have successfully lost weight and kept it off, and much can be learned from their experiences. Most such examples involve a turning point, where the person recognizes they have a problem or unmet need, and then makes a deep commitment to change behavior. The examples almost always confirm the value of the Stages of Change model described in Step 3, showing that people may stay in the contemplation stage for years before moving into action, and that maintenance is the hardest stage of all.

MORE DETAILS

Case example: Sue, part 2

Sue took the message from Vaillant's book *Aging Well* to heart. She knew that she had been neglecting herself and realized that time was passing and the only way she would have the kind of life she dreamed of was to take action. She decided to learn the basics about diet and exercise, and the pitfalls expected when a person tries to change, and she wrote down the reasons she wanted to make the effort: "1. avoid diabetes and crippling joint problems. 2. feel more confident about myself at work and socially. 3. Stop obsessing about weight and diets - find my realistic weight range and stick to it." Sue joined a weight loss group for support and the regular weigh-ins, then (after 6 months) decided she could do it on her own with only occasional support from her physician and close friends.

Now 33-years-old and 20 pounds lighter, Sue feels like a new person. Larry left her a year ago when she started spending time with friends who enjoyed walking and camping in the mountains. She is now dating a man who enjoys food and movies, and also loves being outdoors with Sue and their friends. She is making $10,000 more a year than two years ago, as a manager, and is considering a career change – maybe to something related to travel or event planning.

She has learned to monitor her size (often by how her clothes fit, confirmed by weighing herself periodically) and to strengthen her resolve and renew her commitment to lifelong healthy behavior each time her weight begins to creep up to the upper level of her chosen range. Her proudest accomplishment – and she no longer hesitates before taking some credit for the good things that happen in her life – is she got her mother to join her in a Yoga class, and they both now find excitement and pleasure in planning and preparing healthy and delicious meals. Her mother has lost 30 pounds and is off all diabetes medicine. Sue's blood pressure is normal and her knee hardly ever bothers her. Life is, indeed, good.

Success stories

Sue's story, a composite of several actual people, is not a pipe dream. Even people who fail to achieve their initial weight loss goal often feel very good about what they have achieved. In *Rethinking Thin* author Gena Kolata follows the progress of several obese subjects participating in a University of Pennsylvania weight loss research study. Kolata concludes that, even though few of the research subjects met their weight loss goals after two years, they all "say they have changed because they joined the study and the change was for the good."

(One of the male subjects did lose 15% of his initial weight and kept it off). Here are some examples:

- A man: "I think we all agree it's been a fascinating two years, an almost transforming two years. I lost weight; I gained some of it back. I think I have a good idea of what I can realistically accomplish, which is a lot different than what I thought two years ago."

- A woman: "Eating without thinking – that had been her habit, says Graziella Mann. But no more. ... Now, Graz says, she can't imagine eating so reflexively, and her food choices have changed." Graz, who lost 11 pounds and weighs 212, concludes "I may not be that poster child for dieting, but I am very happy. ... I'm much healthier."

- A man: "Jerry Gordon is a changed person, too. He knows portion sizes; he reflexively estimates the calories in every bit of food he sees. ... And he exercises regularly, walking and using the StairMaster he has at his house. 'It sets a certain tone for a healthy lifestyle,' he says. 'It makes a big difference in your attitude if you can say, "I'm exercising every day and maintaining some kind of control and discipline."' Jerry remains fat. 'Will I ever reach a normal weight? No,' he says. 'That's not going to happen. But I'd say I'm definitely happier.'"[1]

We can learn a lot from our failures and successes, and can learn and be inspired by the success stories of others. This is the idea behind the National Weight Control Registry (nwcr.ws), where over 5000 people who have lost significant amounts of weight and kept it off for over a year tell their stories. The participants lost at least 30 pounds (average weight loss 70 pounds) and kept it off for an average of six years (sometimes for decades). Here is a description of the Registry from their website:

"The National Weight Control Registry (NWCR), established in 1994 by Rena Wing, Ph.D. from Brown Medical School, and James O. Hill, Ph.D. from the University of Colorado, is the largest prospective investigation of long-term successful weight loss maintenance. Given the prevailing belief that few individuals succeed at long-term weight loss, the NWCR was developed to identify and investigate the character-

istics of individuals who have succeeded at long-term weight loss. ...
Detailed questionnaires and annual follow-up surveys are used to
examine the behavioral and psychological characteristics of weight
maintainers, as well as the strategies they use to maintain their weight
losses."
The participants in this registry lost their weight in a wide variety of ways, but
there were some commonalities in how they kept if off:

"The key [according to James Hill] is exercise. 'Activity becomes the driver; food restriction doesn't do it. The idea that
for the rest of your life you're going to be hungry all the time –
that's just silly.' People in the registry get an average of an hour of
physical activity every day, with some exercising for as much as 90 minutes a day. They also keep the fat in their diet relatively low, at about 25
percent of their calorie intake. Nearly all of them eat breakfast every
day, and they weigh themselves regularly. 'They tell us two things,' Hill
says. 'The quality of life is higher – life is better than it was before.' And
'they get to the point with physical activity where they don't say they
love it, but they say "It's part of my life." ... I think you pay the price
for having been obese and you have to do a lot of activity to make up
for that.'"[2]

Dr. Judith Beck's book *The Beck Diet Solution* includes statements from peo-
ple who were successful in losing weight through her program (see Chapter 13
for more details). Here is some of their wisdom:
"I now know ...
- I can control my eating if I plan in advance what I need to do and if I practice
  what I need to say over and over to myself.
- When I'm tempted to eat something I shouldn't, I need to pull out my list that
  contains all the reasons I want to lose weight.
- Just because I'm hungry doesn't necessarily mean I should eat.
- Cravings always go away, and there are things I can do to make them go away
  faster. I don't have to give in to them.

• Eating a reasonable breakfast and lunch is important so I won't overeat at night.

• If I don't follow a nutritious diet, I'm more likely to cheat.

• I have to make more time for dieting and exercise.

• I have to prepare in advance for sabotaging thinking.

• I need to sit down and eat slowly and notice every bite – every time I eat.

• If I eat something I shouldn't, it's just a mistake. It doesn't mean I'm hopeless or bad. I don't have to make a bigger mistake by continuing to eat whatever I want for the rest of the day.

• I have to put my needs first sometimes.

• It's okay to say no to people who offer me food.

• I have to watch out for fooling myself. Every single time I put food in my mouth it matters.

• I need to give myself credit every time I do what I'm supposed to do.

• If I regain weight, I can go back to using the skills I learned to lose it – every time.

• I can do it! I have the skills now. I know how to do it, and I'll have these skills forever."[3]

There have been numerous published reports of successful weight loss and maintenance. For example, in July 2007, *The Today Show* (NBC) featured women who had lost significant weight and kept it off. Their stories appeared in the August 2007 issue of *Good Housekeeping* magazine in a featured article entitled "Half My Size – No surgery, No fad diets – how 7 women lost a total of 1,062 pounds, and kept it off." The women used various methods to lose the weight, but all described a "turning point" when they made a commitment to follow through with their plan to lose weight, focus on health, and get off the roller-coaster. The turning points in the article involved a dire obesity-related medical prognosis or medical crisis for self or loved one, awareness that an important life goal requires weight loss, or an encouraging interaction with a friend or physician. Based on the seven success stories, the article summarized some principles:

- Don't be your own worst enemy – hide tempting snacks and don't keep bad-for-you foods in the house.
- Stay strong – write down triggers that result in overeating so you can "defend yourself" with alternate healthy foods or activities.
- Get moving – 30 minutes of even moderate exercise a day.
- Eat slower – take longer to prepare, heat, defrost or even chew your food.

Book stores and magazine racks are full of such lists and similar advice, especially in January every year. In general, almost any diet or weight loss group can work if the person sticks to it long enough. It all boils down to coming up with your own, individualized plan that you believe in and are willing to follow long-term. The suggestions in this book are meant to spark your creativity and get you going. The details are up to you.

Chapter 8

Step 8: Consider your family and social network

WHAT YOU NEED TO KNOW

We live embedded in a network of relationships, and the nature of these relationships has a profound effect on how we think, feel, and act. The more we are conscious of how these other people affect us, the more control we will have over our own life. Staying in regular contact (if not in person, then at least by phone or email) with people who are working to have healthy habits reinforces our own efforts, and theirs, too. Seeking counsel from a qualified therapist may be necessary to overcome negative family relationships, because simply cutting off contact from family rarely works in the long run and improved relationships are often possible. We certainly cannot change other adults, but we can learn to respond differently to the pressures of family patterns.

MORE DETAILS

One of the most powerful, and underutilized, tools in psychiatry is social network theory. In this chapter I will draw on some of the findings that relate directly to success, or failure, in implementing a weight management plan.

Stress buffering and support

We all live embedded in a network of other people, some of whom exert a negative influence, some a positive influence, and some neutral. The size and shape of the network is important. A large network (at least 25 people) composed of multiple groups of people (five groups of five, say) who are connected to you, but not to each other, is perhaps the ideal configuration when it comes to one of the main functions of a social network: stress buffering.

For example, the five groups may represent immediate family, co-workers, church buddies, neighbors, and basketball buddies. If a major stress comes along, such as losing your job, you also lose one of your network groups, but you still have four others to provide support and distraction, and even concrete assistance if needed. On the other hand, if you only had two groups in your network, say work and family, then all the stress from losing your job would fall on you and your immediate family. There would be little opportunity in that scenario for support or distraction.

This simplistic, concrete illustration should at least give you an idea how important other people and groups of people can be in your life. The takeaway message is that we would do well to nurture and even expand the number of contacts in our lives to increase the potential stress-buffering capability of our network. We can also strive to add more supportive people, as well as individuals who might become allies and co-travelers in our journey toward better health and positive aging.

Another aspect of a social network we can partially control is to minimize our contact with negative people (such as someone who puts us down, goads us to eat or drink too much, is jealous, etc.). This can be done in a variety of ways depending on specific circumstances, and should not be done cruelly, lightly, or without help from a trusted counselor or therapist. The overall goal is to make our social network into a support system. A support system is a collection of people who provide us with emotional, material, and inspirational help and encouragement. As a member of such a system, we are expected to reciprocate, and provide support to others in the system. Our being needed and being useful, in turn, gives our own self-worth a boost. It is a win-win arrangement.

Social networks and being overweight

In 2007, an article appeared in the *New England Journal of Medicine (NEJM)* with the title "The Spread of Obesity in a Large Social Network over 32 Years."[1] The same day the article was published it made front page news. No previous research had focused so intensively on "the obesity epidemic" as a social network phenomenon. The main finding of this elaborate study was that friends have a highly significant influence on our weight, specifically whether we become obese. The effect of friendship was surprisingly large and exceeded the influence of siblings and spouse (whose influence was also significant).

The effect on weight of a friend becoming obese was measured over time and distance, and it was evident that it was the nature of the friendship (mutual and same gender) that exerted the influence, not proximity or mere acquaintanceship. Neighbors who were not friends, and people who were not held in esteem by the research subject, had no impact. The cause of the influence, which works for weight loss as well as weight gain, was thought to be a sharing of ideas – about what is a desirable weight, about food, about health-related choices. The authors concluded that "the psychosocial mechanisms of the spread of obesity may rely less on behavioral imitation than on a change in [a person's] general perception of the social norms regarding the acceptability of obesity."

The study, federally funded and carried out by researchers from Harvard and University of California, has opened up the possibility that weight is at least as much a function of psychosocial factors as it is biological factors. The editorial in the NEJM accompanying the article put it this way:

"As the article by Christakis and Fowler [the researchers] shows, ... networks, in this case those that pertain to social influence, may have just as strong an impact on the development of obesity as the otherwise strong genetic effects. The role of links and connections does not stop here. In the past few years, we learned that network effects increasingly affect all aspects of biologic and medical research, from disease mechanisms to drug discovery. It is only a matter of time until these advances will start to affect medical practice as well, marking the emergence of a new field that may be aptly called network medicine."[2]

A *Time magazine* article about the research concluded:

"Fowler and Christakis say that the contagion-effect should hold just as much for weight loss as it does for weight gain. 'I would hope this influences individuals to get friends and families involved in decisions about health,' Fowler says. After all, he says, a weight-loss plan may be more effective if the people closest to you are on board. And, if you're successful, your good health will help others achieve a healthy weight too. The impact extends not just to your friends, it turns out — but also to your friends' friends, and even to their friends. ... Helping one person lose weight can have a snowball effect through an entire social network."[3]

Other research shows that having supportive people in your life makes a difference in maintenance of weight after an initial loss. For example, an article in the *Journal of the American Medical Association* (March 12, 2008; lead author Laura Svetkey) describes the outcome after 30 months of people who lost an average of 19 pounds through diet and exercise (during the first six months of the study). One group of research subjects was contacted twelve times per year by a counselor who offered encouragement; the people in this group regained almost nine pounds less than those in a group who had no such personal contact. Overall, 71 percent of the 1700 study volunteers maintained at least some weight loss over 30 months. Additional research shows that having a supportive spouse (or significant other) helps maintain weight loss, but a negative partner (for example, one who tempts you with junk food) can sabotage the results.

Family systems

An important subset of our social network is our family system. Family systems are unique in that they exert a multi-generational influence on how we are raised, how we develop, whom we marry, how we raise our children, and what kinds of habits of thought and behavior we adopt.

Family patterns of behavior are powerful and sometimes hidden from plain view. Objectively studying your own multi-generational family in order to better understand the individuals and the patterns is the beginning of a process called "differentiation." The late Murray Bowen, M.D., described this process in many books and articles over the past several decades, and his ideas are kept alive and evolving at the *Bowen Center for the Study of the Family* at Georgetown University. Their web site has a section describing Bowen theory in some detail, and is worth a visit (go to the site at *www.thebowencenter.org/index.html* or do an Internet search for "Bowen Center for the Study of the Family").

Becoming more "differentiated" involves becoming more in charge of one's own life, while still maintaining intimate connections with family members. As one learns how to be more of an autonomous individual in one's own family, and therefore less emotionally reactive to the negative patterns in the family system, one also becomes more able to make and stick to a rational plan for self-improvement. I will conclude this section with a case example:

John, a 36-year-old computer engineer, husband, and father of three children younger than ten, felt confident and in charge of his life, except when he traveled to Boston twice a year to visit his parents and sister. He would feel anxious and irritable for weeks before the trip, and he and his wife, Sally, would argue, it seemed, over nothing. He barely noticed that his eating, normally not a problem, became excessive and compulsive in the weeks before such a visit, during the visit, and for weeks afterward, when he would be alarmed at his five pound weight gain and vow to go to the gym and start a diet.

However, over the years, the ten pounds a year he picked up around the two visits "home" exceeded the five pounds he was able to get rid of through dieting and exercise. It seemed like a vicious cycle, a classic yo-yo situation, and, at 250 pounds, he felt ever more discouraged and tempted to just drop out of his losing battle of the bulge. Yet, his wife and children clearly deserved better, even if he didn't feel deserving. He hated failure, and this fight with himself over food was draining him of confidence, energy and even enjoyment of eating. He now dreaded going out to eat, because all he could think about was what he could and couldn't order.

Finally, depressed and on the verge of marital failure, he saw a therapist who happened to be trained in family systems therapy. The therapist showed John and Sally how to draw diagrams of their multi-generational family systems, and each would take turns talking about family patterns, some of which became clear to them for the first time. John's father, for example, was attentive to John's sister Ellie (who was unemployed and living off handouts from her parents) and practically ignored John, asking only perfunctory questions about his job and children. John's mother, on the other hand, made a huge fuss over John and seemed to thrive on his visits. She expressed this mostly by cooking his favorite comfort foods and insisting they go to his and her favorite Boston restaurants. His parents really did not communicate with each other, Ellie and her mother seemed to dislike each other intensely, and Sally and the kids felt pressured to be helpful, be quiet, or be the center of attention. They did not find these visits relaxing in the least, and Sally had her own issues to deal with when they also visited her parents and siblings twice a year.

The therapist gave John a "homework" assignment that emphasized ways to change his behavior when he visited his parents and sister in Boston. John and Sally both had input into the assignment and agreed to try something different. The same old pattern from the past was clearly not helping anyone!

John and Sally visited John's family three times during the course of a year and a half of therapy, and based on what they learned in the therapy sessions they both now could see how powerful and anxiety-ridden the patterns they had taken for granted really were. Following the plan (homework) developed in therapy, John changed his behavior during the 2nd and 3rd visits to Boston.

He asserted himself more with his mother, and insisted on spending time alone with his father and, separately, his sister. These changes were not so blatant as to cause disruption, but the relationships began shifting in subtle ways. John's parents talked to each other more, Ellie decided to spend more time outside the house (John helped set her up with a support group in Boston which also took into consideration her interest in art), and John, Sally and the kids spent some time on their own enjoying Boston. When he felt anxious during an interaction with his family, John reminded himself of the mantra he learned in therapy: don't attack; don't defend; stay connected.

The most remarkable change, to John, was he no longer ate compulsively before, during and after the visits, and, with renewed confidence and energy, found he could actually follow a sensible and permanent healthy plan for eating reasonably and getting regular exercise. By the second year of therapy, he began *losing* weight at the rate of five to ten pounds per year. He even found, now that he was not obsessed with dieting, that he enjoyed eating more than he had in a **long** time. This dawned on him in a dramatic way when John, Sally, and his parents (Ellie agreed to stay with the kids at home) began going to their favorite Boston restaurant twice a year and enjoying the process for the first time in recent memory.

Chapter 9

Step 9: Learn about alcohol, drugs, and addictive behavior

WHAT YOU NEED TO KNOW

This step is one of the most important, and is the one most often ignored or de-emphasized in the weight management literature. If you do not drink, use recreational drugs, or take prescription drugs, read this chapter anyway. I suspect you know someone who does.

MORE DETAILS

The addiction model for overeating

Overeating does not fit a formal disease model, and it does not fit the addiction model very well, either. Unlike addiction to a psychoactive substance (alcohol, for example), eating ordinary food does not itself alter one's will or voluntary behavior, so putting more food in one's mouth continues as a conscious and voluntary act. Drinking more alcohol, on the other hand, impairs higher brain function and actually does result in loss of self-control: "Man takes a drink. Drink takes a drink. Drink takes the man."

People can be addicted to certain *behaviors* which activate powerful reward systems in the brain, such as gambling and thrill seeking, but eating food is a normal process that all of us must do. For most of us it would be a stretch to label our eating behavior addictive, even though we may feel "out of control." (Occasionally, brain abnormalities result in impaired ability to resist impulsive and addictive patterns of behavior, and in extreme cases this faulty "wiring" may lead to a tendency to overeat).

Overeating and addictions do have some things in common, however, especially in the way many people overcome the problem. In the treatment of addictions, *abstinence* from the substance or behavior is usually the goal, which of course could not apply to overeating. But many techniques used to treat addiction, that tap the power of will to help the person with the addiction remain abstinent, also are helpful to people who overeat:

- making the problem more manageable by approaching it one day at a time and one step at a time;
- teaching new ways of thinking over time;
- offering group and individual support; and
- encouraging changes in environment and people (eliminating enablers and triggers).

Because there are similarities, some people do find viewing their overeating as an addiction helpful and successfully use this model to lose weight and keep it off. Some have found it helpful to view certain types of foods (for example, sugary deserts) as substances they are "allergic" to. If this kind of reframe works for you, use it.

Alcohol

Alcohol consumption is double trouble for weight management. It clouds your consciousness, weakens your will, and decreases your impulse control. It also is a major source of calories. So, if you plan to drink, be sure you take control of how much and under what conditions you do so. For example, two glasses of beer may be fine, but not if part of the process is munching on peanuts. Also, light beer may be a lot better for your plan than full bodied ale.   The calorie content of alcoholic drinks varies widely, and should be a factor in what you choose to drink, and how much. Alcohol itself contains seven calories per gram, almost as much as the nine calories found in a gram of fat and nearly twice that in a gram of protein or carbohydrate. Add fat-filled or sugary mixers, and the calories can reach 500 per drink. Search the Internet for "calories in alcoholic beverages" for more detailed information.

In her book (*The Beck Diet Solution*), Dr. Beck recommends eliminating spontaneous (non-planned) eating and spontaneous drinking. Both how much and what you eat and drink should be detailed in your personal weight management plan. If you drink, she recommends that you "drink slowly so it'll last longer. As soon as you've finished your drink, order a no-calorie beverage, so you won't be tempted to order another alcoholic beverage."[1]

If you believe alcohol might be contributing to your weight gain, experiment with going alcohol-free for three months. After not drinking for three months, you may discover your mind is clearer and body in better shape than you have experienced in a long time. Consequently, you may find planning to lose weight even easier, and your confidence may increase. You can then make a decision as to whether and in what way to include alcohol in your future.

Other drugs

Other recreational drugs, such as marijuana, also affect judgment and ability to stick to a plan. The same advice for alcohol applies here, except calories are not directly a factor. Daily marijuana smoking can be harder to give up than regular alcohol use, but the results after three months "on the wagon" may pleasantly surprise you.

Self-medication

One way one can sabotage his or her healthy living plan is by "self-medicating" with alcohol or other psychoactive substances. This is usually just a pseudoscientific excuse for drinking and drugging, and should be nipped in the bud. If the underlying problem for which one is self-medicating is truly significant, then s/he should see a qualified health professional to get it tended to.

Prescription drugs

It is important to realize that prescription drugs can make weight loss more difficult, especially psychotropic drugs such as antidepressants, anti-psychotics, and mood stabilizers. These should be discussed in detail with the prescribing physician and any weight loss plan modified accordingly.

Screening tests

Two common screening tests for problem drinking are the CAGE[2] and the RAPS4[3] (answering "yes" to any one of the questions is cause for further assessment):

CAGE[2] (Cut down, Annoyed, Guilty, Eye-opener):

1. Have you ever felt you should cut down on your drinking?
2. Have people annoyed you by criticizing your drinking?
3. Have you ever felt guilty or bad about drinking?
4. Have you ever had a drink first thing in the morning to steady your nerves or to get rid of a hangover?

RAPS4[3] (Remorse–Amnesia–Perform–Starter):

1. During the last year have you had a feeling of guilt or remorse after drinking?
2. During the last year has a friend or a family member ever told you about things you said or did while you were drinking that you could not remember?
3. During the last year have you failed to do what was normally expected from you because of drinking?
4. Do you sometime take a drink when you first get up in the morning?

Chapter 10

Step 10: Create a plan and routines

WHAT YOU NEED TO KNOW

Now that you have clear goals and are armed with the basic knowledge of the important factors affecting weight management, it is time to commit to a specific plan. Plans involve sub-goals, or steps, and are much more specific than goals and a general commitment. Not everyone needs to write a detailed plan, but doing so will not hurt and may make a big difference in your ability to follow through realistically.

MORE DETAILS

Creating a plan

Most goals must be broken down into small, manageable steps (some call these steps "objectives" or "sub-goals") before they can be attained. This involves planning, much of which may be done outside our conscious awareness. For example, we may set a one-time goal to visit brother Tommy in London next November. The steps (each of which has sub-steps) might be:

- check with Tommy re dates he is home;
- renew passport;
- arrange coverage at work and time off;
- put aside $100 per pay period in a travel account (shop and go out to eat less!);
- find the best flight deal;
- arrange for placement of dogs and cat;
- see if Anna might want to come, too;
- check weather in London and plan travel wardrobe; etc.

Whether or not the steps are written down in a formal way, they still exist and will take time, thought, and energy.

A similar sequence of steps for a goal of weight loss might be:
- write down all the reasons I chose this goal and refer to list often (place it on refrigerator and bathroom mirror, and carry in wallet);
- pick desired target weight or range (one year from now I will weigh five pounds less than I do now);
- estimate for a week how many calories I take in per day;
- become familiar with the basic nutritional guidelines (Step 6 in this book) and start shopping with these in mind;
- list the high calorie foods I can easily learn to do without and keep these out of the house;
- list the ones I can easily cut down on and only eat them as a treat or reward;
- plan to eat only at set times (three meals and a light evening snack);
- eat only while sitting and eat from a plate (a small plate is best);
- list ways I can distract myself when I feel hunger pangs, or crave something; refer to list when tempted to overeat;
- list useful reframes when I am tempted to snack while watching TV or at night; refer to list as needed;
- drink water with meals and often;
- spend less time with Jim who is always eating, and more time with Bill who likes to walk and hike;

- visit Mom only once a month and stay for only two hours (I always eat too much at her house!) – talk with her on the phone every other day to compensate for fewer visits;
- do not buy sugary treats or snacks for home or work;
- do not take others' candy when offered at work;
- consult with a qualified personal trainer 2 or 3 times to come up with a realistic (and fun!) strength-building exercise routine I can do at home using inexpensive equipment (weights, bands, ball, step, etc.);
- make a time and place at home to exercise three times a week while listening to radio or podcasts;
- exercise spontaneously by parking farther away, walking instead of driving, using stairs, and moving more at work;
- take a walk for at least 20 minutes five times a week (do it in mall if weather is bad);
- re-check calories taken in per day after three months;
- weigh myself weekly and adjust plan accordingly, but try to lose no more than one or two pounds per month;
- avoid thinking or saying I am "on a diet" (because this is the way I want to eat and exercise for life);
- never think of what I am giving up, only what I am adding to the quality of my life.

The example above lists a sequence of steps that a particular person might choose. It does not represent an ideal or model plan. Every plan should be unique to the needs and interests of the person to whom it applies.

Setting priorities

If we have five important goals, there may be more than 100 steps involved in making them happen. We might feel overwhelmed at the prospect of deciding to do all these steps. So, we may need to order them in terms of priority and when they must be done. The ones most in line with our personal mission statement (if we choose to have one; see Step 1) should have the highest priority. Adding a new goal might involve eliminating an older one. The list should be dynamic and change as our circumstances, accomplishments, and priorities change.

The payoff for a weight management goal and plan is long-term. It might take years to fully realize the benefits, one of which is that the plan itself will eventually become more or less automatic and not require much conscious effort. As you think about your priorities, and your plans to accomplish various life goals, it will be important to reaffirm the importance of weight management and you may need to recommit to this goal on an annual basis.

The best way to ensure your plan does become a natural part of your lifestyle, and something you adhere to consistently, is to make most of the steps routine. For example, brushing teeth before bed is not something most of us think about – we just do it, and feel strange if we don't. Similarly, if we shop, eat, and exercise pretty much the same way every day or week, it will soon seem effortless. It is important to remind ourselves that the discomfort of changing behavior is temporary, and must be endured if we are truly going to change our lifestyle.

PART TWO

Chapter 11

Empower yourself to change your behavior - easy action steps to get you started

This chapter consists of things to do, or exercises, that I have labeled **easy action steps**. These are an important part of preparing yourself for lifelong weight management and some contain information not found in Part I of this book. Many call for action on your part besides just reading and thinking. Writing and using the Internet utilize brain circuits that simply reading and thinking don't engage. The brain is a wonderful organ, and one of its wonders is how different types of experience activate different brain pathways which interact with each other in a synergistic way. So, if an exercise calls for writing, please get out pen and paper and give it a try; and please don't worry about grammar, spelling or penmanship!

EASY ACTION STEPS YOU CAN TAKE NOW TO PREPARE YOURSELF FOR CHANGE

Step 1: State a reason to change your behavior.

1. List the health concerns you have that may be related to weight, BMI, or waist circumference.

2. Use the Internet (see http://www.nhlbisupport.com/bmi/) to calculate your own BMI and see which category you may be in (e.g., normal weight, overweight, obese). Also, measure your waist circumference and write these figures down where you can refer to them later. Check out this website: http://www.nhlbi.nih.gov/health/public/heart/obesity/lose_wt/risk.htm

3. On the Internet, search "personal mission statement" and "goal setting." Play around with what you find (many use simple fill-in-the-blank forms that help you create a written list in a short time period). Think about this process for the next week and try it again at least a week later.

4. Write a paragraph expressing your positive and negative reactions to the process of setting goals in general, and health-related goals specifically.

5. Write a goal for weight management for yourself, using your most important personal incentives and desires in the statement. How is this goal different from a New Year's resolution for you?

6. Do you identify with any part of Sue's story (case example)? Briefly list how you may have similar, and different, issues.

7. Write a paragraph or two about social stigma and how you feel it applies to Sue's life, your own life, and our culture.

Step 2: Choose a realistic weight range.

1. Write a paragraph describing your feelings about the term "overeating." Identify both positive and negative implications of the concept (as defined in this chapter) for you.

2. Estimate your current calorie needs, based on your age, gender, height and weight. One easy way to do this is to go to www.mypyramid.gov, click on MyPyramid Plan and follow the simple directions. You will get nutritional and caloric intake suggestions based on the latest government dietary guidelines. I suggest you do this several times as you progress in your resolve to modify the way you eat.

3. Check out this website to help you choose a desirable weight range: www.halls.md/ideal-weight/body.htm (Steven Halls, the site designer, is a radiologist in Alberta, Canada) or do an Internet search for "ideal weight" or something similar.

4. When you are ready for more detailed information about your calorie-in/calorie-out situation and needs, keep a diary of everything you eat for a typical day and use the program found on www.mypyramid.gov in the MyPyramid Tracker section (simple registration required). Check the site out to see how it works before you start the diary.

Step 3: Learn about "willpower" and self-change.

1. Answer the questions: How relevant do you feel biological factors (that you cannot directly control) are to your efforts to manage your weight? Roughly, what percentage of your eating do you feel is determined by your free will (less than 20%, 20% to 40%, 40 to 60%, 60% to 80%, more than 80%)?

2. Practice substituting "I won't" every time you are tempted to say "I can't." How does this make you feel?

3. Write a paragraph or two about how you feel about taking full responsibility for your decisions. Mention both the positives and negatives.

4. Think about, and then list, a few examples from your life when you really wanted something and made a strong effort to get it. Include successful efforts as well as failures.

5. Practice thinking like an optimist as described in this chapter (that is, when something good happens, think "I did that. I do that kind of thing in many ways. It's a permanent part of who I am." But when a bad thing happens, think "It was the situation. And that situation was unique. Anyway, it'll be different next time.") How does it feel? Is this something you can learn to do more of? Why would you choose not to? Be honest with yourself. No one else needs to see or hear what you are thinking.

6. List some examples of how you have been influenced in your eating decisions by marketing, advertising, and what you have been exposed to. Do you think it would be possible to change any of your beliefs about food in general, and about specific foods? Would it be possible to ever change your feelings about these foods?

7. Before reading the rest of this step, write a few sentences describing how you feel about weight management. Is there any way you could re-word (reframe) your statement to be more positive and still be factual and realistic? If you used "I should" or "I need" in your statement, try substituting "I want." How does that feel?

8. Think of a situation in your life when your thoughts, feelings and actions were NOT congruent, or in alignment. Now, think of a situation where they WERE in alignment. Write a paragraph about how the two experiences compared.

9. Think about two or three areas of your life (e.g., some specific issue you have with your health, career, family, etc.) that involve change and apply the stages of change model. Which stage do you think you are in for each area you chose?

10. Answer the question: What stage are you in with regard to weight management, and what would have to happen for you to enter the next stage?

11. If you have ever had the experience of relapse, write a paragraph about both the positive and negative aspects.

Step 4: Learn how to manage stress.

1. List three sources of stress in your life, and how you usually manage the discomfort and soothe yourself. Be thorough and honest in your descriptions.

2. Write about episodes in your life when you have binged (rapidly gulped large quantities of food and feeling sick, guilty, or ashamed afterward). Include times when you weren't even aware that is what you were doing, but now suspect you were.

3. List all of your comfort foods, and briefly describe when and how you eat them (include what you eat while watching TV or at a movie theater). Note when you do this without conscious awareness, without paying full attention to the food you are eating, and also when you do it as part of a reasonable eating plan. If you wish, try to pinpoint why a particular food gives comfort (past memories, associations, etc.).

4. Do you ever eat out of boredom? What else could you do when you are bored that would be better for you in the long run?

5. Look up "mindfulness" on the Internet and read about it. Is there a way you can easily incorporate this practice in your daily life? How might it apply to eating?

6. Respond to each of the methods of relaxation mentioned in this chapter (silence, breathing, music, reading, nature, beauty, meditation, relaxing exercise, sexuality) by stating whether you have used it and to what effect. Are there any of these you would like to do more of? Are any of them unappealing? What other methods can you list?

7. Use your willpower to give love and attention to a significant other at a time when you feel you need love and attention. How did it feel to do this, and what was the outcome?

Step 5: Guard against "willpower fatigue."

1. Think about how willpower fatigue affects you. Give an example (preferably in writing) of a time you got sidetracked from a difficult task or project because you ran out of steam. What were the consequences? Did you recover your willpower and commitment after a break? How might willpower fatigue affect your plan to eat less and exercise more?

2. Write a paragraph or list describing what your patterns of resistance to change are. What do you characteristically do when you are ambivalent about something?

3. Write about an example from your life when you did successfully follow-through with a difficult change. How might you transfer what you learned to better managing your weight?

4. If you are "stuck" and not making progress with some aspect of your life, write a "legal brief" arguing forcefully both sides of the case (for and against change).

5. Talk to a trusted friend or therapist and ask them for their honest thoughts about ways you might be sabotaging yourself.

6. Think about how you handle anger, and whether you ever take it out on yourself. Write a paragraph on how you will turn anger from a negative into a positive.

7. Ponder the statement "not making a decision is making a decision." How do you feel about it? How might it apply in your life?

8. Write a few sentences about times you have "rewarded" or "indulged" yourself by eating or drinking too much, and what the positive and negative consequences were.

9. Review Chapter 5 and pick the three forms of resistance to change that you have experienced. Write a few sentences about each one and how it affects your life.

10. After you have read all of the *easy action steps* in this chapter, make a list of the ones you are least likely to do. Any step you are avoiding is probably one that touches a sensitive nerve and may therefore be an important one for you to do. If you do it in spite of your resistance, you will have certainly exercised your willpower!

Step 6: Learn the basics about diet and exercise.

1. Weigh yourself once a week for a month and keep a record. How do you feel about this? Do you think weighing regularly makes a difference in how you view your lifestyle and what choices you make? What other techniques could you use to monitor progress?

2. Schedule an hour to go to the grocery store and shop for food by reading labels and generally following the nutrition guidelines in this chapter. Write a paragraph about how the experience was for you. How often would you have to shop this way before it would become easier? What shortcuts do you think you could take to make health conscious shopping easier? Would paying for a nutritionist to do this with you a few times make a difference (note: nutritionists take into consideration your food preferences)? Try it.

3. If you have not already done so, use the Internet to take the Portion Distortion Quiz: http://hp2010.nhlbihin.net/portion/.

4. Make a list of ways you can incorporate more energy expenditure from physical activity into your daily routine (spontaneous exercise, non-exercise activity, and formal exercise). How can you arrange to stand, walk, and use stairs more?

5. Pick a pleasant time and place and take a walk for 45 minutes. Don't worry about how fast you go. Later, you can map out a 2 – 3 mile route and see how much of it you can cover in 45 minutes. Invest in a well fitting pair of walking shoes.

6. If you have any concerns about your physical ability to exercise, make an appointment with your doctor or other qualified health professional to get an objective evaluation and recommendations. Physical therapists can be wonderful sources of this kind of information (seeing a physical therapist may have to be "ordered" and overseen by your doctor).

7. Consult a recommended personal trainer and/or Yoga instructor to help you fine-tune your exercise plan.

8. If you smoke or take diet drugs, write about your experience, including pros and cons. Consider seeing a qualified professional to discuss the health implications, including weight gain, of stopping the tobacco or drugs.

9. Experiment with changing your attitude toward a variety of healthier foods. Notice that how you think about the food makes a difference in how much you enjoy it. Some people refer to vegetables as "rabbit food," for example, which guarantees they will not enjoy them. Does "healthy" have a positive or negative connotation to you? Make a conscious effort to change the way you think about food so that you place more value on healthy choices.

10. Talk with a friend about becoming a walking or biking buddy.

11. Visit a food store that emphasizes local, seasonal, and organic food [note: organic foods are more expensive and not necessarily more healthful than non-organic foods; but they are worth checking out and are probably better for the planet].

12. Watch the movie Super Size Me (2004).

Step 7: Learn from others' experience.

1. Write a short story ("case example") with yourself as the main character. Include how you have changed your lifestyle and what you will be doing two to five years from now.
2. Go to the website of The *National Weight Control Registry* and explore the personal stories and research findings [www.nwcr.ws].
3. Think about the people you know and have known. Have any of them successfully changed their lifestyle in a healthy direction? Have any lost weight and kept it off? If so, think about (and/or ask about) how they did it. How does this information affect you?

Step 8: Consider your family and social network.

1. Describe or, better yet, diagram your social network in terms of groups of people you see regularly and how they are or are not connected with each other.
2. Think of an example of "stress buffering" from your life where your social network helped you get through a tough situation.
3. List all your close same-gender friends, even ones who live far away. Now, try to remember which of them gained (or lost) weight during the course of your friendship. Do you see a pattern that confirms the finding that friends influence changes in your weight (and vice versa)?
4. Look for and briefly describe two or three relationship patterns in your family of origin (including at least three generations).
5. How do you usually feel, both positively and negatively, when visiting your own parents or extended family? What emotional age do you feel like during the visits?
6. What about those visits (that you could control) could be different?
7. How does your family affect how you eat and exercise?

Step 9: Learn about alcohol, drugs, and addictive behavior.

1. Think about how the concepts "disease" and "addiction" are used in your family and peer group. Answer the question: How does the use of these words help or hinder you in your efforts to take control of the quality of your life?
2. If applicable, describe a time when you or a family member has struggled with alcohol or drugs. How did you resolve the issue?
3. Think about the concept of self-medication and whether you have tried it. What was the underlying problem and what did you do about it?
4. Read the CAGE and RAPS4 screening tests and honestly ask yourself the questions. Even if they don't apply to you, if they do apply to a friend or family member, you might be affected.

Step 10: Create a plan and "routines."

1. State a weight management goal and write at least five specific sub-goals that would constitute a weight management plan for you.
2. Pick a trusted friend, family member or therapist and talk about how this process felt for you. Share your goal and plan with this person and get their response. Do this with another person if you wish.
3. After reading Chapter 13, think about the cognitive-behavioral techniques described and pick the top three you are tempted to try. Make notes about how you might implement the techniques.

Chapter 12

Research on weight management

This chapter consists of summaries of some important research findings related to diets, causes of weight gain, the process of losing weight, and the health effects of weight gain and loss.

Research on diets

A widely reported government-sponsored study from Stanford University, published in 2007, compared four diets and found modest weight loss of 3.5 to 10.5 pounds after one year of follow-up (311 overweight/obese premenopausal women were randomly assigned to follow one of four diet books, receiving weekly instruction for two months, plus a follow-up session in month ten).[1] The Atkins diet had the best results (Zone, Ornish and LEARN were the other diets), and the lead researcher emphasized that the main messages from the research were: 1) twelve months is a very short time to assess a diet; 2) even with a lot of help, research subjects had a very difficult time adhering to the diets; 3) although subjects lost a relatively small amount of weight (they were 50 – 100 pounds overweight), there were health benefits (lower blood pressure, lower cholesterol, improvement in insulin metabolism); 4) the authors do not recommend the Atkins diet based on this study, because they think women in that group lost weight primarily because they ate fewer carbs (especially less refined sugar, white breads, and high fructose corn syrup), not because they ate a lot of fat.[2]

There have been many other attempts to study the effectiveness of diets, but few have been as well-designed as the Stanford project. Essentially, all of the other research had similar findings: people have a great deal of difficulty sticking to a diet; the weight loss tends to be modest; no particular diet shows a significant advantage; and most people regain the weight after stopping the diet. People who go on serial diets tend to have weight that goes up and down, and over time this yo-yo effect has negative health consequences.

Unfortunately, research on something as complex as nutrition is limited in what it can tell us. One reason is that in order to control variables, usually only one main outcome is being studied. So, for example, if a study shows almonds might help improve your lipid profile, that study says nothing about the effect of almonds on your weight management program. (Nuts, in general, are nutrition-ally good, but also are very calorie dense, so eating them is a trade off. They should be in your diet, but as a substitute for other high-density foods that are not so nutritious.) It is a good idea to treat any reported study as highly prelimi-nary until it has been replicated several times by unbiased experts. As a rule of thumb, if a book or article touts a specific product (food, food additive, potion, drug, exercise device) and it is likely the manufacturer funded the "research" behind the product, take it with a large grain of salt.

Bio-psycho-social factors in weight gain and loss

Although common overeating (and under-exercising) is neither a disease nor an addiction, modern medicine teaches that all health-related states are caused by a combination of biological (such as genetic), psychological (like stress) and social (such as friendships) factors. Research on overeating shows that there are complex neuro-chemical, environmental (especially the availability of cheap, energy-dense food in large portions), and behavioral explanations.

The brain has at least two areas, or systems, that affect our eating: a survival-based ("homeostatic") system activated by energy deficits, and a pleasure-based ("hedonic") system activated by the presence of palatable food. Both of these systems are affected by multiple factors and appear to function semi-independently from each other.[3]

The pleasure-based brain system affecting eating behavior is similar to the pleasure seeking part of the brain that drives some addictive behavior. Therefore, some research on addiction also may help us understand overeating better. It teaches us that the prefrontal cortex (the "higher" part of the brain) is the area that overrides the pleasure-seeking and impulsive areas of the brain, and that the neurotransmitter GABA is a key brain chemical that communicates this inhibition to the "lower" part of the brain that is responsible for craving. Neuroimaging studies (e.g., functional MRIs) have shown that in addicts, after 3 to 18 months of abstinence, the brain actually changes back to its pre-addiction state to a large degree, and the craving at this point becomes minimal.[4]

So, it may well be that what I am calling willpower resides in the prefrontal cortex, that GABA is involved in our ability to control our impulses and cravings, and that after we *consistently* practice new eating patterns the old "overeating" patterns become weaker or extinguished. Much more research is needed in this area.

Other research suggests that complex brain functions, including conscious decision-making efforts, interact to regulate our eating behavior, and that the overwhelming abundance of large portions of highly appealing food in our society can easily overwhelm our natural tendency to stop eating when we have had enough.[5] One author who does research in rats on the effects of food choice on overeating concludes that the term "obesity by choice" describes how many of us become overweight. It is true that both rats and people tend to overeat when they have more food choices readily available.[6]

As discussed in Chapter 6, research by Dr. Levine has shown that our baseline activity level (NEAT, or non-exercise activity thermogenesis) has a significant effect on our weight, and that a sedentary lifestyle clearly contributes to being overweight.

A federally funded research study, involving over 12,000 people tracked over 32 years, reported in 2007 that social network connections – especially friendship choices – may influence weight gain even more powerfully than genetics. Other research shows that our relationships affect our ability to maintain a desired weight (see Chapter 8 for details).

Thus, a tendency to gain weight is bio-psycho-social, with psychological, chemical, hormonal, volitional, cultural, and relationship factors contributing. However, unlike coronary heart disease which also has multiple contributing factors (including behavior, or lifestyle), the ONLY way a person can actually gain weight is through the conscious, voluntary act of eating. Except in relatively rare neurological and sleep disorder conditions, the act of eating is done while one is fully awake and in control of one's behavior.

If one were physically restrained from putting food in one's body, as occurred in concentration or prisoner of war camps, and as also occurs in some hospital-based food restriction programs, one would lose weight. It used to be thought that food restriction (or "restrained eating") always results in overeating when the restriction is removed, and this is usually the case, but research shows that *reduced* binge eating and healthier eating habits can also result.[7] Almost all researchers agree that the best results from weight management efforts occur in preventing weight gain, rather than losing weight once it is gained. *Maintaining* a desired weight after a period of weight loss is even more difficult than the weight loss itself.

Biological reductionism

"Biological reductionism" is a form of determinism that is popular in medicine and medical writing today. It is the point of view that your body is a collection of chemicals and physiological processes over which you have little control. In psychiatry, this mode of thinking results in a tendency to prescribe pills for most symptoms and conditions. I think this trend has gone too far in psychiatry and medicine, and is partly fueled by the huge profits over-prescribing has generated for the pharmaceutical industry.

The book *Selling Sickness*[8] makes the point that medical data (such as lipid levels, bone density, and "hyperactivity") are being used to broaden the definition of what is a "disease" so that treatments (usually drugs) can be sold to more and more people who may, in fact, be functionally well. The same thing may also be happening with "overweight," which is not in itself a disease (except for some forms of "morbid obesity").

In her book *Rethinking Thin*,[9] Gina Kolata, a *New York Times* science reporter, agrees that being "overweight" has been oversold as a health problem. She correctly criticizes the hugely profitable "diet industry" for capitalizing on people's belief that they can and should try to change what they weigh. However, she also makes the argument that people have little control over their weight and that, like height, it is mostly biologically determined through a poorly understood interaction of heredity and environment. This argument is an example of *biological reductionism* because it minimizes the role of psychosocial factors that we can individually influence through our intentional behavior, or willpower.

I agree with Kolata that being overweight is not necessarily a medical problem and also agree with her criticism of dieting, but I disagree with her emphasis on how little effect our behavioral choices have on the outcome. For example, she writes, "It must be that free will, when it comes to eating, is an illusion."[10] She throws out the baby "willpower" with the bathwater of self-blame and shame. The problem, as I see it, is not with willpower but with the misuse of it in trying to comply with worthless diet plans and attempting to achieve unrealistic goals.

For some people there is a major genetic and/or biochemical component to their difficulty in maintaining the weight they desire. Ongoing research concerning the roles of leptin, ghrelin, insulin, and many other hormones in regulating body weight and hunger demonstrates that some obese individuals (perhaps as many as 5% or more) may have genetic mutations affecting their ability to control their appetite. Related lines of research indicate there are biological forces that make it difficult for most people to lose weight once it has been gained. Such evidence suggests that once fat tissue accumulates, a system of overlapping neurological and hormonal mechanisms works to prevent it from diminishing. Even so, most of us do have a significant degree of control over our eating and activity level, and this means we have *some* control over what we weigh.

Kolata concludes her book with this statement, which is a bit pessimistic in tone, but also offers realistic hope for people who are interested in taking action toward improving their health:

"The lesson is, once again, that no matter what the diet and no matter how hard they try, most people will not be able to lose a lot of weight and keep it off. They can lose a lot of weight and keep it off briefly, they can lose some weight and keep it off for a longer time, they can learn to control their eating, and they can learn the joy of regular exercise. Those who do best tend to be those who learn to gauge portions and calories and to keep their houses as free as possible of food they cannot resist. The effort, the lifelong effort, can be rewarding – people say they feel much better for it. But true thinness is likely to elude them."[11]

Many people do beat the odds and lose significant amounts of weight, and keep it off, through lifestyle change (see Chapter 7).

Weight loss and health

One of the most intriguing lines of research has to do with the direct effects of losing weight on health status. For example, patients who have stomach-reducing bariatric surgery do better than obese people who don't have the surgery in that they have less diabetes, and their mortality from diabetes (after an average of seven years) is 92 percent less than obese patients who do not have the surgery. Patients who have the surgery also are 60 percent less likely to die from cancer and 56 percent less likely to succumb to heart disease. Additional findings, following patients an average of eleven years post-surgery, show a 30 percent overall decrease in mortality. Patients in these studies lost an average of 14 to 25 percent of their pre-surgery weight.[12]

The exact mechanisms of such health benefits from stomach surgery are not understood. It is interesting that research on liposuction does not reveal similar health benefits. It appears that removing 20 pounds of fat surgically does nothing to improve health status. On the other hand, research shows that there are health benefits in people who lose weight by eating less and exercising more, with even small losses resulting in improved blood pressure, cholesterol, and glucose metabolism. So, pursuing a healthy lifestyle promotes health for most people *even if they don't lose much weight.*[13]

Conclusion

Research on causes of obesity and overeating is expanding rapidly, and that is a positive development. But there are so many different points of view that it can be overwhelming. It is like the four blind men describing an elephant: the first, standing at the trunk, says it is thick and tubular, like a big snake; the second, at the ear, says it is flat like a pancake; the third, at the tail, says it is like a whip; and the fourth, at the side of the elephant, says it is like a huge wall.

With obesity, some researchers focus on the hormonal systems and animal models and conclude weight is determined by overwhelmingly powerful biological mechanisms. The neuroscientists point to the brain as the key element (but have yet to fully explore conscious volition and its pathways). Psychologists and social scientists look at the epidemic, behavioral, and interpersonal components. Physicians and other health-care professionals are more concerned with how to prevent and reverse negative health consequences.

Some research tries to bridge the gaps, but no single study or discipline can encompass the entire problem. My conclusion from all of this is that we are far from having final answers and that all points of view have some validity. My bias – and my chosen "frame" – is to focus on what we, as individuals, can influence. Although much happens in life that is beyond our control, and some are far luckier than others, I insist on believing in free will, because that notion is what gives my life zest. I decide, therefore I am.

Chapter 13 - Advanced techniques for behavior change

Specific Cognitive-behavioral Techniques For Controlling Weight

This chapter describes additional "cognitive/behavioral" techniques for thinking and acting designed to support the implementation of your weight management plan. I introduced the concept of Cognitive Behavioral Therapy (CBT) in Chapter 3, and now will discuss some of the more formal and advanced methods in use today to help people create healthier lifestyles.

Dr. Beck's self-help book

CBT was first introduced as a form of "talk therapy" in this country in the 1950s (in the form of Rational Emotive Behavioral Therapy) by Albert Ellis, Ph.D, and was also made popular by the independent work of Aaron Beck, M.D. (who used the term Cognitive Therapy). Aaron Beck's daughter, Judith Beck, Ph.D., has written a self-help book applying CBT to weight management: *The Beck Diet Solution.*[1]

Although Dr. Beck's program requires participants to choose their own "diet" (a primary one and a backup diet) from any of the numerous nutritionally valid ones available, and refers to her clients as dieters, I prefer to avoid the word "dieter" and, instead, think of the readers of this book as people committed to attaining and maintaining a chosen weight range that works for them.

Regardless of the terminology used to describe the program and its clients, the CBT principles and methods can be very helpful. Aaron Beck, MD, writing in the Foreword to his daughter's book, summarizes the kinds of erroneous thinking ("sabotaging thoughts") people who have difficulty losing weight often use:

- rationalization (*It's okay to eat this because ...*);
- underestimation of consequences (*It won't matter if I eat this*);
- self-deluding thinking (*Since I cheated a little, I might as well eat whatever I want for the rest of the day*);
- arbitrary rules (*I can't waste food*);
- mind-reading (*My friend will think I'm rude if I don't eat her cake*);
- and exaggeration (*I can't stand being hungry*).

Here are some additional examples from Dr. Judith Beck:

- all or nothing thinking (*either I'm completely on my diet or I'm off my diet*);
- negative fortune telling (*Since I didn't lose weight this week, I'll never be able to lose weight*);
- overly positive fortune telling (*It's okay if I just estimate the amount of food I'm supposed to have instead of measuring it – I'll still lose weight*);
- emotional reasoning (*I feel like I just have to have something sweet right now*);
- unhelpful rules (*I can't waste food*);
- justification (*I deserve to eat this because I'm so stressed out*);
- exaggerated thinking (*I have no willpower*).[2]

Cognitive Behavioral Therapy teaches people to become aware of silent self-talk (the "little voice in your head") and to recognize harmful or false statements (sabotaging thoughts) such as "I am a failure" or "I am starving!" Such thoughts are humorously referred to as "stinking thinking." In the course of therapy or reading about CBT, people learn to replace such negative self-talk with positive messages (thoughts Beck calls "helpful responses"), such as "one slip does not make me a failure" and "I am having hunger pangs, but do not need to eat right now." This technique is similar to reframing, which was discussed in Chapter 3.

Judith Beck's *Diet Solution* is a detailed forty-two day step-by-step program which addresses these "crucial factors:"

- Choose a nutritious diet.
- Create time and energy for dieting.
- Plan what and when you're going to eat.
- Seek support.
- Deal with disappointment.
- View overeating as a temporary problem that you can solve.
- Cope with hunger and cravings.
- Eliminate emotional eating.
- Give yourself credit.[3]

Participants (i.e., readers of her book) spend the first two weeks doing such activities as writing down the advantages of losing weight, thinking about what you're eating before putting it in your mouth, practicing eating only when seated, eating slowly and mindfully, eating only to mild fullness, doing spontaneous exercise daily and planned exercise three times a week, creating time and energy so you can implement your plan, practicing hunger tolerance, and learning how to overcome cravings.

For the next four weeks they actually go on the diet they chose, weighing themselves weekly (at least weekly weighing continues indefinitely in this program). Dr. Beck believes that "any reasonable diet will work for you if you have the right mindset."[4]

Some of the lessons during this phase include monitoring eating, sticking to a detailed "eating plan" ("cheating" is reframed as "unplanned eating"), learning to say "Oh, Well" to disappointment and unfairness, dealing with discouragement, recognizing thinking mistakes, resisting "food pushers," deciding about drinking alcohol, eliminating emotional eating, solving problems, reducing stress, and dealing with a weight loss plateau.

Sections of the book discuss the most common problems people face while trying to control their weight, such as dealing with environmental "triggers" for overeating; handling eating out, vacations and special occasions; and distinguishing among the different types of hunger (true hunger, desire, and craving).

Dr. Beck states that hunger is generally a poor guide to follow in how much you eat (you should stick to an eating plan, instead).

A key component of the program is for each participant to select a *diet coach* from among their friends, family members, or other potentially supportive people. The functions of the coach are to provide external motivation and encouragement, help with building confidence, and help with problem solving. Joining an organized support group or even finding a weight loss support group on the Internet are options.

Beck summarizes the main principles of her program this way:

- Eating is not automatic. You *can* learn to take control.
- Many situations trigger thoughts about eating, but there are techniques that you can learn to avoid or minimize these triggers.
- When you encounter a trigger, your thoughts determine whether you act in a productive way that strengthens your *resistance muscle* or in an unproductive way that strengthens your *giving-in muscle*. [emphasis added]
- Responding to your sabotaging thoughts is a skill that you can use for your lifetime to keep of excess weight permanently.[5]

There is little direct research on the effectiveness of this book or program, but Dr. Beck mentions a study in Sweden that found "people enrolled in the Cognitive Therapy program lost an average of 18 pounds over ten weeks of treatment. (Meanwhile, people on a waiting list to get into the program didn't lose any weight.) ... When the researches re-evaluated study participants a year and a half after treatment, their average weight had continued to drop whereas the average weight of the people on the waiting list had increased."[6]

Beck's book was reviewed online by a spokesperson for the *American Dietetic Association* ("the nation's largest organization of food and nutrition professionals"), Lisa Dorfman, MS, RD, CSSD, LMHC, who wrote: "I would recommend this book to a yo-yo dieter who feels she has tried every diet but just keeps gaining the weight back. This book is not a crash diet but instead helps develop eating behaviors for life. The reader is told to set realistic goals (like a five-pound weight loss) and to celebrate each time that goal is reached, rather than immediately setting a goal of 30 pounds. The importance of slow, steady weight loss ... is emphasized in this book, as is the importance of committing oneself for life and not just quitting once the goal weight is reached."[7]

Other books featuring CBT for weight control

Dr. Beck's book emphasizes the importance of weight maintenance and the acquisition of life-long skills to maintain one's desired "maintainable weight," and recognizes that the biggest problem with long-term weight control is the maintenance phase. Another CBT book, aimed at clinicians rather than dieters, also focuses strongly on the persistent problem of weight regain after initial loss: *Cognitive Behavioral Treatment of Obesity: a Clinician's Guide*.[8] In their individual therapy approach, the authors describe the treatment as occurring in two phases.

Phase One (17 sessions in 30 weeks) focuses on weight loss and Phase Two (seven sessions in 14 weeks) focuses on weight stability. The three main elements of the total program are:

• Drawing a distinction between weight loss and weight maintenance.
• Addressing during the weight loss phase potential obstacles to the acceptance of weight maintenance (i.e., weight stability) as the goal in Phase Two.
• Helping patients acquire, and then practice, the behavioral skills and cognitive responses needed for effective weight control.

As mentioned in Chapter 1, the authors emphasize the importance of patients choosing other personal objectives besides weight loss. In both Beck's program and this program, reminding people why they wanted to lose weight is critically important.

Weight *maintenance* skills follow these principles:

• Successful weight maintenance requires balancing energy intake with energy expenditure.
• Patients need to practice maintaining their weight over a range of circumstances (e.g., vacations, ill health, times of stress).
• Weight needs to be regularly monitored and evaluated.

- Changes in weight are almost always due to a change in energy intake or activity level, or both (exceptions are pregnancy, some illnesses, and some medications).
- Correcting for changes in weight involves either a change in energy intake or a change in expenditure, or both (changing intake is the more potent of the two).
- There is evidence that those people who maintain an active lifestyle are most successful at weight maintenance.
- Significant weight change must be spotted and promptly addressed.
- Once weight has returned to the target range, there needs to be a further correction of energy intake or expenditure (or both) to maintain the new weight.[9]

One of the authors of *Cognitive Behavioral Treatment of Obesity*, Christopher Fairburn, has also written a self-help book for people who have a problem with binge eating, *Overcoming Binge Eating*.[10] He emphasizes a CBT approach to this problem and some research supports its effectiveness.

Additional comments on CBT and weight management

The books highlighted in this chapter are consistent with the approach I have been advocating, and may be helpful for those of you who want to delve further into Cognitive Behavioral Therapy. The treatment can be very effective, but requires willingness and ability to precisely and rigidly adhere to a long series of very detailed exercises.

Before you commit to one of these programs, there is a lot you can do on your own, armed with the information in this book. You can do brief "experiments" (which, when successful, become new healthy habits) to overcome fear of hunger and cravings and learn that you can distract yourself from such impulses in healthy and creative ways. For example, if you get hungry prior to a planned meal time, you can practice using self-talk ("this hunger feeling is temporary and just a remnant of my old habit of snacking" and "brief bouts of hunger do not mean I am being deprived" and "I will eat in an hour and can find something else to do in the meantime") and distractions such as calling a friend, going for a walk, or doing a chore to get it out of the way, to replace the old (snacking) behavior with new (non-eating) behavior. After a short while (usually a matter of weeks), the old habit-pattern may fade away and cease to be a problem, except for occasional relapses.

The **Easy Action Steps** in this book (Chapter 11) are experiments, and doing them will likely help you progress toward your goal(s). Do them and see what the results are – that is what an experiment is. Success with such experiments adds up to increased confidence and establishment of new and healthier patterns.

Initially, having an eating plan, with your personal goals clearly specified and written objectives (or steps), may be necessary. Monitoring what you eat, even writing down calories, may be helpful for a while. Paying attention to calories is not difficult now with so much information available on labels or the Internet (as long as you pay close attention to portion size), and precise calorie counting is seldom needed in the long run. Also, you will learn your new eating patterns well enough to pace yourself by eating less at times to make up for eating more at other times. At some point, the rules can be relaxed or modified so long as the previous eating pattern does not return. The course of progress will not be linear, and there will be relapses and plateaus.

Extra effort will be needed to deal with times of extra temptation, such as parties, holidays, when alcohol is consumed, and in the presence of certain people who constantly eat or offer food. You can learn to be more assertive with people who offer food, can physically leave the area if needed, and can also plan to eat more at one meal (e.g., if it is a special occasion) and less at others to compensate.

Learning what foods to eat more or less of, or add or subtract from meal planning, will involve trial and error over time, but can be an adventure and add excitement and fun to the process. "Diets" are characterized by limitation, restriction, and deprivation, but lifelong weight management should not be dreary or unpleasant in any way.

So often, our responses to foods are accompanied by automatic thoughts that occur almost subconsciously when a food or food group is presented.

"Ugh, I don't like vegetables" or "fruit is boring" or "the sweeter, the better" or "I crave French fries and nothing else will do" are all self-defeating thoughts that WE CAN CHANGE. CBT is all about the power of thoughts and behavior and how we can exert conscious control over them. Are vegetables really yucky? Is sweet really that great? Is all fruit boring? When you learn to think positively about fruits and vegetables, for example, and less lovingly about sugar and butter, healthy eating becomes fun.

Chapter 14 - Summary and conclusion

We have a big say in how well we do, physically and emotionally, as we age. Most of the factors that predict positive outcome in later life are at least partially under our control. We can learn to think optimistically and can reverse "learned helplessness."

Willpower (and "won't power"), by which I mean conscious volition and self-empowerment, is necessary for making desired changes, but tapping the power of our will is not always easy. Biological factors play an important role in weight management, especially when we try to lose weight we have gained. Prevention, keeping the pounds off in the first place, or at least stopping the weight gain trend, is extremely important.

Taking full responsibility for our decisions is clearly something we do at times, and do often where food is concerned. But behavior change can be difficult and take a while to feel natural and effortless. Slow and steady wins the race.

Some basic knowledge about food and exercise (including non-exercise activity) and a few fairly simple skills are necessary for us to adopt a healthy lifestyle. Following the ten steps outlined in this book will give you a running start, especially if you do the **easy action steps** in Chapter 11.

Going on a temporary "diet" seldom helps and often contributes to our failure to take full responsibility for our lives. Successful lifestyle change does not require that we feel deprived. "Diet pills" are not very effective and cause problems of their own. Eating and moving are, and should continue to be, great sources of joy and socialization.

Choosing a realistic weight range as a goal is important, as is knowing roughly how many calories we take in and how many we expend in our daily life. Having a realistic set of high-priority goals that we believe in can help us focus our effort and stay on track with our plan to manage our weight. For many, weighing regularly is a valuable part of monitoring progress and preventing setbacks.

With practice, we can change our patterns of thinking so that thoughts, emotions, and actions are congruent, or in alignment. We can change our preferences for food and activity in ways that support a healthy (and happy) lifestyle.

Knowing the predictable stages of self-change can help us maintain focus, keep our expectations in line with reality, and prevent us from falling into common traps.

It is normal to get tired of working on a self-improvement plan and to find excuses to take time off. Honest self-evaluation can help us pinpoint specific areas of resistance-to-change and willpower fatigue, and this self-knowledge may be sufficient to allow us to get back on track. If not, finding a compatible counselor or therapist may be indicated.

Learning healthy, easy, and effective ways to reduce stress will help us stay focused on our long-range plan.

Cognitive Behavioral Therapy (CBT) techniques can be readily adapted to aid us in our weight management program. The basic skills are easy to grasp and master, but advanced skills may require help from a book, a coach, or a therapist.

Creating and utilizing a supportive social system will help us stay on a healthy path. Our friends may even affect how much we weigh more than our genes do. Family-of-origin issues can pull us back into patterns of behavior we are trying to change. There are ways to learn to be more in control of our lives while still staying connected to the healthy parts of our family system.

Use of alcohol, drugs, and self-medication can sabotage our plan. There are ways to gain control of the situation, but denial is not one of them. Prescribed medication also can affect weight and should be carefully evaluated.

Changing one's health-related behavior occurs in stages, must be based in reality, takes willpower, education, practice, supportive friends (and family), and persistence, and it helps to have some kind of plan with goals. There is no magic and it can be difficult, but becomes much easier the more you do it.

I wish you well on your lifelong journey to health and happiness! Please let me know how you are doing. Contact me through my website.

Charles Goldman, MD
www.weightmanagementforyourlife.com

Acknowledgments

My initial interest in writing this book was sparked by discussions, sometimes heated, with my friend and colleague Peter Swanson. At first we took opposing positions: he emphasized that being overweight is the result of our genes and biological systems and there is little we can do about it; I argued that what we *decide* to do about our eating and exercising makes a huge difference, not just in our weight but in our overall health. As the discussions continued, with emails flying back and forth over several months, we both studied the research and read books on the topic of weight management. Eventually, each of us moderated our views and, though perhaps not in total agreement, came up with a balanced and research-based set of conclusions. I decided to write them down, and the ideas evolved further as I learned more about the subject and as others became actively involved in the discussion. The result of this evolution was *Weight Management for Your Life*.

My wife, CheChe Goldman, son and daughter-in-law Andrew and Heather Goldman, and step-daughter Anna Hamilton have provided invaluable feedback and support. I deeply appreciate their patience and constancy. I am extremely grateful for the editing suggestions and input from friends and colleagues Ted Wachter, Jan Collins, Rose Butterfield, Harriet Wall, and several others.

Notes

Introduction

1. Vaillant G: *Aging Well*. Little, Brown & Company, Boston, 2002.
2. Vaillant, pp. 210–213; emphasis added

Chapter 1. Step 1: State a reason to change your behavior

1. Minsky M: *The Emotion Machine – commonsense thinking, artificial intelligence, and the future of the human mind*. Simon & Schuster, 2006 (hardback edition). p. 191.
2. For example, workout guru Bob Greene on *the Oprah show* (NBC November 28, 2007).
3. There are many easy-to-use tools on the internet for calculating your BMI (Body Mass Index) – all you need to know is your height and weight; for example, see www.nhlbisupport.com/bmi/. The formula is BMI = (Weight in Pounds / (Height in inches) x (Height in inches)) x 703.
4. Abdulla SM, et al: The association of differing measures of overweight and obesity with prevalent atherosclerosis. *J Am Coll Cardiol.* 2007 Aug 21; 50 (8): 752–9.
5. Cooper Z, Fairburn CG, Hawker D: *Cognitive Behavioral Treatment of Obesity*. New York: Guilford Press, 2003.
6. *Cognitive Behavioral Treatment of Obesity*, p. 6.
7. The Global Obesity Series, www.theworld.org/?q=taxonomy_by_date/1/20080101.

Chapter 2. Step 2: Choose a realistic weight range

1. Fairburn and Brownell (editors): *Eating Disorders and Obesity, 2nd edition*, The Guilford Press, 2002; Chapter 106, page 588.

2. Beck J: *The Beck Diet Solution*. Birmingham, Ala: Oxmoor House; 2007.

3. Kolata G: *Rethinking Thin*. Farrar, Straus and Giroux, 2007. p. 209.

Chapter 3. Step 3: Learn about "willpower" and self-change

1. NPR.org, 4/12/2007.

2. Kolata G: Rethinking Thin. Farrar, Straus and Giroux, NY, 2007, p. 42

3. References for Baumeister and Seligman studies: Can You Increase Your Willpower? by Ansary T *(http://encarta.msn.com/column_willpower_tamim-home/Can_You_Increase_Your_willpower_tamimhome.html);* and Tighten Your Belt, Strengthen Your Mind, by Aamodt S and Wang S (*New York Times*, April 2, 2008).

4. Kolata, p. 170.

5. Kolata, pp. 128–129.

6. Kolata, p. 184.

7. Decision-Making Deficits and Overeating: A Risk Model for Obesity. *Obesity Research* 12:929–935 (2004).

8. There is much evidence that changing your thinking through willpower can even change the structure of the brain itself. For example, see Begley S: *Train your mind, change your brain*. Ballantine Books, 2007.

9. Do an Internet search for "Prochaska and DiClemente" and/or "stages of change" for more information.

Chapter 4. Step 4: Learn how to manage stress

1. http://www.washingtonpost.com/wp-dyn/content/article/2007/07/01/AR2007070100431.html (July 2, 2007).

2. Wansink B: *Mindless Eating:Why We Eat More Than* We Think. Bantam Books, 2006.

3. www.news.cornell.edu/stories/jan07/food.mood.sl.html, January 23, 2007.

Chapter 5. Step 5: Guard against "willpower fatigue"

1. Martin Binks, PhD, Director of behavioral health, Duke University's Diet and Fitness program; NPR.org, 4/12/2007.

2. Baumeister RF: Yielding to Temptation: Self-Control Failure, Impulsive Purchasing, and Consumer Behavior. *Journal of Consumer Research*, volume 28 (2002), pages 670–676; also, Vohs KD, et al: Decision Fatigue Exhausts Self-Regulatory Resources. Feb 15, 2006 www.gsb.stanford.edu/facseminars/events/marketing/pdfs%202006/2006_02-15_Vohs.pdf.

Chapter 6. Step 6: Learn the basics about diet and exercise

1. Nestle M: Eating Made Simple. *Scientific American*, September 2007, p. 60.

2. Pollan M: *In Defense of Food*. Penguin Press HC, The; 1 edition (January 1, 2008)

3. Fairburn and Brownell (editors): *Eating Disorders and Obesity, 2nd edition*. The Guilford Press, 2002; Chapter 106, page 590.

4. www.news.cornell.edu/stories/jan07/food.mood.sl.html, January 23, 2007.

5. www.news.cornell.edu/stories/Nov05/popcorn.pigs.ssl.html, Nov. 9, 2005.

6. *US News and World Report* 3/20/05. Also, *Sugar Shock* by Bennett C and Sinatra S (Berkley Trade, 2006).

7. theworld.org, global obesity series, 1/1/08.

8. www.health.gov/dietaryguidelines/dga2005/document/html/executivesummary.htm. See also www.health.gov/dietaryguidelines/dga2005/document/pdf/brochure.pdf and www.iotf.org/popout.asp?linkto=http://www.cdc.gov/nccdphp/dnpa/obesity/.

9. Kolata, p. 52.

10. Chair Today, Gone Tomorrow. *Nutrition Action Health Letter*, April, 2008. Also, http://www.mayoclinic.org/news2005-rst/2630.html.

11. www.dukenews.duke.edu/2000/09/exercise922.html, Sept 22, 2000.

Chapter 7. Step 7: Learn from others' experience

1. Kolata G: *Rethinking Thin*. Farrar, Straus and Giroux, NY, 2007. pp. 215–218.
2. Raeburn P: Dropping weight…and keeping it off. *Scientific American*, September 2007, p. 67.
3. Beck p. 13.

Chapter 8. Step 8: Consider your family and social network

1. Christakis NA and Fowler JH: The Spread of Obesity in a Large Social Network over 32 Years. *NEJM* Volume 357:370–379 (July 26, 2007, no. 4);
2. Barabasi A: Network Medicine — From Obesity to the "Diseasome." *NEJM* Volume 357:404–407 (July 26, 2007, no. 4)
3. Blue L: Obesity is Contageous, Study Finds. *Time*, July 25, 2007.

Chapter 9. Step 9: Learn about alcohol, drugs, and addictive behavior

1. Beck, pp. 220–221.
2. Dhalla S, Kopec JA: The CAGE questionnaire for alcohol misuse: a review of reliability and validity studies. *Clin Invest Med.* 2007;30(1):33–41.
3. This test is called the *Rapid Alcohol Problems Screen (RAPS4)* and was developed by ARG Senior Scientist Cheryl J. Cherpitel, Dr.P.H., R.N. The name is also an acronym for Remorse–Amnesia–Perform–Starter. For technical information see the following: Cherpitel CJ: A brief screening instrument for problem drinking in the emergency room: the RAPS4. *Journal of Studies on Alcohol* 61, 447–449 (2000).

Chapter 10. Step 10: Create a plan and "routines"

No notes

Chapter 11 - Empower yourself to change your behavior - action steps to get you started

No notes

Chapter 12 - Research on weight management

1. Gardner CD, et al: Comparison of the Atkins, Zone, Ornish, and LEARN Diets for Change in Weight and Related Risk Factors among Overweight Premenopausal Women. *Journal of the American Medical Association.* 2007;297:969–977 (March 7, 2007);

2. Your Health – Stanford Study Weighs In on Popular Diets. NPR, *Talk of the Nation Science Friday*, March 9, 2007, interview with Christopher Gardner, MD, www.npr.org/templates/story/story.php?storyId=7806284.

3. Lowe MR, Levine AS: Eating motives and the controversy over dieting: eating less than needed versus less than wanted. *Obes. Res.* 2005 May;13(5):797–806.

4. Lemonick M: How we get addicted. *Time*, 7/5/2007.

5. Rolls ET: Understanding the mechanisms of food intake and obesity. *Obesity reviews* (2007) 8 (Suppl. 1), 67–72.

6. Tordoff MG: Obesity by choice: the powerful influence of nutrient availability on nutrient intake. *Am J Physiol Regul Integr Comp Physiol* 282: R1536-R1539, 2002.

7. Wardle J: Eating behaviour and obesity. *Obesity reviews* (2007) 8 (Suppl. 1), 73–75.

8. Moynihan R and Alan Cassels A: *Selling Sickness*, Nation Books, 2006.

9. Kolata G: *Rethinking Thin*. Farrar, Straus and Giroux, 2007.

10. Kolata, p. 155.

11. Kolata p. 217.

12. Reference: *Washington Post*, August 23, 2007, p. A12.

13. Kolata, pp. 210–211.

Chapter 13 - Advanced techniques for behavior change

1. Birmingham, Ala: Oxmoor House; 2007.

2. Beck, pp. 195–196.

3. Beck, p. 24.

4. Beck, p. 19.

5. Beck, p. 32.

6. Beck, p. 20.

7. www.eatright.org/ada/files/BeckDiet.pdf.

8. by Cooper Z, Fairburn CG, Hawker D. New York: Guilford Press, 2003.

9. Cooper et al, p. 168-169.

10. New York, Guilford Press, 1995.

INDEX

Made in the USA
Lexington, KY
18 May 2012